A Time to Embrace

Why the Sexual and Reproductive Justice Movement Needs Religion

Rev. Debra W. Haffner

Religious Institute

Religious Institute
21 Charles Street
Suite 140
Westport, CT 06880

Printed in the United States of America

ISBN 978-0-9855949-5-4

For more information, visit www.religiousinstitute.org

TABLE OF CONTENTS

ACKNOWLEDGMENTS

Many people contributed to the development of A *Time to Embrace: Why the Sexual and Reproductive Justice Movement Needs Religion.*

The Religious Institute is indebted to the religious leaders and executives of sexual and reproductive health and justice organizations who gathered on April 16, 2015, in Washington, DC, for the National Colloquium on Faith and Sexual and Reproductive Health and Justice to discuss the status of faith in the sexual and reproductive health and justice movement and who created many of the recommendations in this white paper. Their names appear on page 59. We are so thankful for their collaboration with the Religious Institute and the important work for sexual and reproductive justice each of them does in the world. We are especially grateful to Linda Bales Todd, Rev. Rob Keithan, Rev. Harry Knox, Patricia Miller, Rabbi Dennis Ross, Aimée Thorne-Thomson, and Lisa Weiner-Mahfuz, who provided comments on the draft of this white paper.

More than forty-five people responded to our requests to complete the surveys that inform this report. The Religious Institute is appreciative of their time, their candor, and their wise comments. A list of the survey respondents is found on page 60.

Members of the Religious Institute staff and board played important roles in the development of this white paper. The Religious Institute's 2014–2015 Scholar in Residence Drew Konow helped organize the colloquium, compiled much of the research for this report, worked on the surveys, and drafted sections of this report. Deputy Director Marie Alford-Harkey participated in the colloquium, drafted the theological section, and provided wise counsel and review. Blanca Godoi provided extensive administrative support. I am also grateful to Religious Institute board members Rev. Dr. Miguel De La Torre and Rev. Dr. Marvin Ellison for their extensive reviews of the draft paper. I am so appreciative of Alex Kapitan's magical editing and Alan Barnett's design work.

This white paper was written during my fortieth year of work in sexual and reproductive justice and my twelfth year of ordained ministry. I am grateful to all of my mentors and colleagues along the way, especially those with whom I worked at the Population Institute, the US Public Health Service, the Center for Population Options (now Advocates for Youth), the Sexuality Information and Education Council of the United States, and for the past fifteen years, the Religious Institute

I dedicate this report to the late Dr. Douglas Kirby, dear friend and long-term colleague, who I wish were still here to have provided his warm counsel and questions as I wrote it.

The Religious Institute acknowledges with great appreciation the David and Lucile Packard Foundation, especially project director Lana Dakan and Director of the Population and Reproductive Health Program Tamara Kreinin, for their belief in the need for this white paper and the financial support that made it possible.

— *Rev. Debra W. Haffner*

EXECUTIVE SUMMARY

Renewing the engagement of religious leaders and people of faith is essential to the progress and long-term success of the sexual and reproductive health and justice (SRH and RJ) movement. Although mainline and progressive religious leaders played a central role in helping to legalize and increase access to contraception and then abortion services during most of the twentieth century, today religious leaders on the Right are more visible in public policy debates, and in many states and in Congress they have been increasingly influential in curtailing reproductive rights. The fact that a majority of people in the United States support legal abortion while a majority also believes that abortion is not morally acceptable demonstrates the need to develop a faith-based approach to closing the morality/legality divide and increase support for reproductive health services. It is time for the sexual and reproductive health and justice movement to once again embrace the influence of religion in the United States to further sexual and reproductive justice for all.

RELIGION IN THE UNITED STATES

The United States is one of the most religious countries in the world. More than three-quarters of people in the United States identify with a religion,[1] and more than half attend worship at least once a month.[2] Attacks on reproductive rights have been the most virulent in the South and Midwest, where more people claim religious affiliations.[3] Religious practice has a special salience to many African American and Latino populations, who make up an increasing proportion of Protestant and Catholic churches.[4]

Religious affiliation helps shape US perspectives on sexuality, contraception, abortion, and LGBTQ issues. Contrary to popular belief, people across

religious traditions in the United States express support for sexual rights, sexuality education,[5] and contraception.[6] Majorities of all religious groups—with the exception of white evangelical Protestants—believe that abortion should be legal in all or most cases.[7]

"We must include faith leaders in an authentic, sustained way. Connecting with people of faith is essential to our goals. We cannot advance sexual health and rights without it."

—Colloquium participant

HISTORY OF FAITH ENGAGEMENT

Protestant and Jewish clergy were centrally involved in the early days of the birth control movement. In the 1930s, religious denominations passed the first resolutions in support of birth control. In the 1940s, Planned Parenthood formed its first National Clergyman's Advisory Council. In 1946, more than 3,000 clergy signed a statement against religious opposition to birth control provisions. In the 1950s, clergy successfully protested Roman Catholic hospitals' decisions to restrict birth control services, and in the 1960s, clergy were a driving force in the movement to secure access to legal abortion.[8]

Fifty years later, religious voices continue to influence public policy about abortion and contraception, although it is often the religious voices that oppose sexual and reproductive rights that have been the most visible in the media and most influential in policy debates. The 2014 Supreme Court decision *Burwell v. Hobby Lobby Stores, Inc.* has invigorated new attempts to deny sexual rights and reproductive health care. The aftermath of the Hobby Lobby decision and the proliferation of so-called Religious Freedom Restoration Acts (RFRAs) on the state level demonstrate the need for mainline and progressive religious leaders to claim and define "religious freedom." When religious arguments are used to deny people rights, religious voices that support justice are an essential part of the response.

THEOLOGICAL GROUNDING

There are many strong public health arguments for supporting sexual and reproductive health services that are well known to secular sexual and reproductive health and justice organizations. There is also ethical and religious grounding for supporting sexuality education, contraception, and abortion that must be widely disseminated and understood. The values articulated by the reproductive justice movement and an intersectional understanding of economic, social, and sexual and reproductive

---

ABOUT TERMINOLOGY

The term "sexual and reproductive health and justice" as well as the abbreviations SRH and RJ are used throughout this report to refer to organizations, professionals, and activists involved in the sexual and reproductive health (SRH), pro-choice, reproductive rights, and reproductive justice (RJ) movements. Many organizations define themselves by only one of these frames, and some do not address broader sexuality or economic issues. "SRH and RJ" is used in this report to broadly include organizations working to protect family planning and abortion services, as well as the movement as a whole. It is also used by the Religious Institute as an umbrella term for such issues as sexuality education, contraception, abortion, and equality for lesbian, gay, bisexual, transgender, and queer (LGBTQ) people. The framework of justice resonates deeply within diverse religious traditions, and its use is intentional for establishing relationships with religious leaders and faith communities. See page 12 for more on these and other key terms used in this white paper and their definitions.

Among many sexual and reproductive health and justice organizations, the term "women" is used to describe people who can become pregnant, use hormonal contraception, have babies, or have abortions. The Religious Institute recognizes that sexual and reproductive health and justice is not just a women's issue, although women are among those who are most impacted. As we attend to the important ways that gender and reproductive health intersect, particularly how women's moral agency and sexuality are demeaned in public debates about abortion, we must also recognize the unique needs of transgender women, transgender men, genderqueer people, intersex people, and others with marginalized gender identities within the realm of sexual and reproductive health and justice. Whenever possible, this report utilizes inclusive language to refer to people who can become pregnant.

"Far Right" is used to describe those in organized movements that use religious language to denigrate sexual and reproductive health, rights, and justice. Over the years, this minority of religious voices has been identified by such names as the Religious Right, the Moral Majority, and the Right Wing. Because religion is often used as a tactic by these organizations, many of which are in fact secular and not religious, we have chosen to follow the lead of the Center for American Progress and identify them as the Far Right.

health issues are crucial to engaging a broader spectrum of faith leaders.

Abortion is morally complex for a majority of people in the United States. Many more people think abortion should be legal than perceive abortion to be morally acceptable.[9] Although almost seven in ten think abortion should be legal, just under half do not think it is a moral option for themselves or their family.[10] The existence of this "morality/legality divide" requires sexual and reproductive health and justice activists and professionals to articulate their work as a moral movement grounded in the moral agency of women, people of color, and other marginalized communities as well as larger social justice efforts. In particular, there is a need to help the US public and lawmakers understand that deciding to have an abortion is a moral decision, that only the person who is pregnant can decide how to respond to an unwanted pregnancy in each particular circumstance, and that it is unethical and immoral to deny people access to life-saving information, education, or safe and timely health care services.

"People of faith are a resource, not an obstacle, to reproductive health and justice. Ignoring the role of faith has weakened our movement."

—*Colloquium participant*

The Surveys

The Religious Institute conducted four surveys with a total of forty-five organizations, denominations, and foundations in preparing this white paper. The Religious Institute surveyed the largest and most influential national sexual and reproductive health and justice organizations; denominations and denominational groups that work on reproductive health advocacy; national organizations that focus on the intersection of faith with SRH and RJ; and foundations that provide support for work on sexual and reproductive health, rights, and/or justice.

One hundred percent of foundations and faith-based organizations and 89 percent of secular organizations responding to the survey agreed or strongly agreed that it was important for the sexual and reproductive health and justice movement to do more to engage religious leaders and people of faith. Table 1 provides a snapshot of some of the key questions by sector.

Secular Organizations

Leaders from nineteen secular sexual and reproductive health and justice organizations responded to the survey. Although most of these organizations reported that they are interested in engaging faith in their work, very few have dedicated resources to doing so. Overall, they do not have staff working on faith, programs that address faith, strategic plans that address faith, articulated values-based visions for their organizations, or a religious leader on their boards of directors. There has been effective work to combat or contain conservative and Far Right religion's negative reach into sexual and reproductive health, rights, and justice issues, and periodically these secular organizations bring a "faith face" to an advocacy issue through a coalition letter or public rally. But few of the organizations have systematically engaged religious leaders or people of faith in their efforts to achieve sexual and reproductive justice. In order to further engage religious leaders and people of faith, leaders of secular SRH and RJ organizations indicated that their organizations would need funding, materials, and training on how to engage religion in the United States.

Denominations

There is a long history of religious denominations advocating for reproductive health. Religious leaders have played a significant role in securing access to abortion and contraception in the United States. Many denominations continue to advocate for reproductive health and rights. Out of the nine denominations or denominational groups surveyed, 77 percent reported that they are moderately to very active on sexual and reproductive health and justice issues. Eighty-nine

Table 1. Survey Highlights

	Secular SRH and RJ organizations	Denominations	Faith-based SRH and RJ organizations	Foundations
Publish materials on faith and SRH and RJ	28%	78%	100%	N/A
Policy statement on faith and SRH and RJ	11%	89%	60%	N/A
Interested in doing more on faith and SRH and RJ	74%	89%	N/A	54%
Think it's important for SRH and RJ field to do more on faith (agree/strongly agree)	89%	Not asked	100%	100%
Work with faith-based SRH and RJ organizations	89%	89%	100%	N/A
Attend worship at least once a month	32%	89%	100%	Not asked

percent include family planning, abortion, and/or reproductive justice in their public policy work. Yet only two denominations have increased their work on these issues in recent years, and many have struggled to maintain their historical commitments to reproductive health. Only the presidents of the most progressive denominations have consistently spoken out for sexual and reproductive health and justice. Denomination survey respondents indicated that they need funding, increased staffing, materials, and training support to do more advocacy work in this area.

FAITH-BASED SRH AND RJ ORGANIZATIONS

The surveyed secular organizations and denominations and their working groups regularly turn to six organizations that work at the intersection of faith with sexual and reproductive health and justice. There are three core organizations—the Religious Institute, the Religious Coalition for Reproductive Choice, and Catholics for Choice—that work exclusively on these issues. Three much larger national organizations—Americans United for Church and State, the National Council of Jewish Women, and the Center for American Progress—have significant programs addressing faith and SRH and RJ issues. These six organizations together have formal networks encompassing more than 15,000 reli-

gious leaders from every US state and have worked to articulate moral frameworks, motivate religious leaders and people of faith, create resources, train spokespeople, and present a progressive religious voice on sexual and reproductive justice issues. The three core organizations together only have fourteen staff people working on domestic sexual and reproductive health issues and are under-resourced for their missions. These organizations have the knowledge and ability to motivate a wide range of diverse religious leaders and people of faith to speak out from a moral perspective in national, state, and local controversies about sexual and reproductive justice. They have contributed significantly to the SRH and RJ movement but are under-resourced for the breadth and depth that is needed.

FOUNDATIONS

The need for funding for work at the intersection of religion with sexual and reproductive health and justice was a consistent theme in the interviews, surveys, and colloquium discussion. Only half of the foundations that were approached responded to the request to complete surveys about their work in religion (a total of fourteen respondents). Although most had made a few faith-based grants, almost 40 percent had not. Foundation leaders overall were likely to have a negative view about the role of religion in securing sexual and reproductive rights. Yet most said that they were likely to fund a faith-based project in the future, and all agreed or strongly agreed with the statement, "It is important for the sexual and reproductive health and justice field to do more to engage mainstream and progressive people of faith and religious leaders."

CALL TO ACTION

This white paper concludes with a call to action based on the surveys, review of the research, interviews, and deliberations at the Religious Institute's National Colloquium on Faith and Sexual and Reproductive Health and Justice. The colloquium participants affirmed that the sexual and reproductive health and justice movement **must articulate a values-based vision and adopt strategies to more fully engage religious leaders and people of faith.** The call to action urges secular and faith organizations to adopt and integrate reproductive justice as central, positioning reproductive health and rights within a larger social movement to empower all people, particularly women of color and low-income women, to have the economic, educational, social, and political power and resources they need to support their decisions about their bodies, sexualities, health, and families.

There is a pressing need to address the morality of sexual and reproductive health decisions; in particular, those committed to sexual and reproductive justice must work to close the morality/legality divide and help the US public and lawmakers understand that abortion is a moral decision. Efforts to destigmatize abortion and change the cultural narrative must involve religious leaders at the outset to fully engage morally complex issues. Together, we must shift the cultural conversation from one of judgment to one of empathy, compassion, and affirmation of people's moral agency. There need to be many more convening opportunities for secular and faith leaders to create joint strategies at national, regional, state, and local levels and to develop trusting, long-term, and sustained relationships.

INTRODUCTION

Renewing the engagement of religious leaders and people of faith is essential to the progress and long-term success of the sexual and reproductive health and justice movement. Although mainline and progressive religious leaders played a central role in helping to legalize and increase access to contraception and then abortion services during most of the twentieth century, today religious leaders on the Right are more visible in public policy debates, and in many states and in Congress they have been increasingly influential in curtailing reproductive rights. The fact that a majority of people in the United States support legal abortion while a majority also believes that abortion is not morally acceptable demonstrates the need to develop faith-based approaches to closing the morality/legality divide and increasing support for reproductive health services. It is time for the sexual and reproductive health and justice movement to once again embrace the influence of religion in the United States to further sexual and reproductive justice for all. This movement must increase its understanding and appreciation of the role of religion in public life and public policy and do much more to create engaged relationships with faith leaders and faith communities.

In April 2015, the Religious Institute convened the National Colloquium on Faith and Sexual and Reproductive Health and Justice, bringing together leaders from national sexual and reproductive health and justice secular organizations, faith-based SRH and RJ organizations, denominations, and foundations. The purpose of the colloquium was to assess the role of religion in the SRH and RJ movement, develop strategies to more effectively engage religious leaders

and people of faith, and make recommendations for greater cooperation among religious leaders, people of faith, and the SRH and RJ organizations. Colloquium participants reached consensus around an overarching vision: **sexual and reproductive health and justice organizations and their funders must recognize and support the involvement of religious leaders and people of faith as essential to meeting their goals.**

There is no question that some parts of organized religion have contributed to profound cultural and personal confusion about sexuality. Organizations on the political right have so effectively used religious leaders to carry their message that there is a widespread misperception that the religious voice is monolithically negative about sexuality and reproductive health and justice issues. For far too long, conservative and Far Right religious voices have dominated the religious discourse surrounding sexuality education, family planning, abortion, and LGBTQ rights. These religious-based arguments must be countered by religious leaders and people of faith speaking out in favor of sexual and reproductive health and justice from historically grounded faith positions. When religious arguments are used to deny people rights, only religious voices that support justice can authentically respond.

This white paper explores the landscape of religion in the United States, the history of religious leaders' involvement in the movement to obtain reproductive rights, religious support for issues pertaining to sexual and reproductive health and justice, current faith-based activities of key organizations, and opportunities to do more to engage mainstream and progressive faith voices. The report ends with a **multifaceted call to action to articulate sexual and reproductive health and justice as a moral movement,** supported by religious leaders and people of faith. Only then can the movement's core commitments to family well-being, women's moral agency, and comprehensive social and economic justice become a reality.

Definition of Terms

Reproductive Justice

According to the organization SisterSong, which created the term: "Reproductive justice emerged as an intersectional theory highlighting the lived experience of reproductive oppression in communities of color. It represents a shift for women advocating for control of their bodies, from a narrower focus on legal access and individual choice (the focus of mainstream organizations) to a broader analysis of racial, economic, cultural, and structural constraints on our power."[11]

Reproductive justice "happens when all people thrive. It will be achieved when all people have the economic, social, and political power and resources to make healthy decisions about our bodies, genders, and sexuality, families and our communities in all areas of our lives.... Peoples' ability to make decisions on their bodies, health, family formation, family support, etc. are affected by the ways in which the health care system, schools, law enforcement, the welfare system, immigration system, and the like see them and interact with them."[12]

Sexual Justice

Sexual justice encompasses the availability of contraception and abortion, HIV/STI prevention, screening and treatment, and the right of all adults to make responsible sexual choices, independent of marital status, gender identity, or sexual orientation. According to theologian Marvin Ellison: "Sexual justice means...honoring the goodness of human bodies and recognizing sexuality as a spiritual power for expressing care and respect through touch. [It] requires recognition of and respect of sexual difference, including diversity of body shape and size, sexual orientation, gender identity and expression, and marriage and family patterns. Sexual justice calls for respect and compassionate care between persons and groups. Fair distribution of social power and goods is also required along with safety, health, and empowerment, especially for the vulnerable."[13]

Social Justice

Social justice refers to the obligation of society to make sure all people can obtain and exercise their rights.

"In religious traditions and groups, the term *social justice* indicates an approach to ethical life in which beliefs and practices support and guide evaluations of and responses to societal, environmental, and cultural conditions. Social justice is differentially identified with religious and philosophical notions of human beings and society, and ideals of compassion, dignity, interdependence, and just relations." Additionally, "social justice is associated historically with the organization of resources and distribution of power."[14]

RELIGION IN THE UNITED STATES

The United States is one of the most religious countries in the world. Religion and spirituality shape our ideals and beliefs, inform our private and communal devotions, and influence our conduct in everyday and sociopolitical contexts, including our sexual and reproductive health decisions and attitudes. Even those who do not adhere to any particular religious community or practice inevitably encounter religion in their friends, neighbors, and communities. Religious beliefs and affiliations affect how people view sexual and reproductive health and justice issues, how likely they are to vote on them, and their attitudes about morality.

THE UNITED STATES IS RELIGIOUSLY ENGAGED AND RELIGIOUSLY DIVERSE

Despite recent media reports about declining religious affiliation, religion remains very important to the vast majority of people in the United States. More than three-quarters (78 percent) report some religious affiliation.[15] There are thousands of denominations and an estimated 350,000 congregations in the United States.[16] A majority (58 percent) of the US population says that they pray every day, with people from most religious traditions reporting daily prayer.[17] Most (92 percent) believe in God.[18] More than half (54 percent) say they attend a religious service regularly (at least once or twice per month),[19] and more than one-third (35 percent) report that they attend worship services weekly.[20]

Diversity is a hallmark of the US religious landscape. Although almost three-quarters (72 percent) of the United States identifies as Christian, there are multiple denominations, beliefs, theologies, sociopolitical perspectives, and practices within US Christianity.[21] Almost half of US Christians (48 percent) identify as Protestant, and almost a quarter (23 percent) identify as Catholic.[22] Within Protestantism, there are many diverse denominations with significant differences in theology, structure, and practice. The Pew Religious Landscape Survey explains: "The Protestant population is characterized by significant internal diversity and fragmentation, encompassing hundreds of different denominations."[23] Among Protestants, 18 percent are white evangelical Protestants, 14 percent are white mainline Protestants, 8 percent are black Protestants, 3 percent are Latino Protestants, 2 percent are Mormon, and 3 percent are other types of Protestants.[24]

Outside of the Christian majority, there are numerous other thriving religions in the United States. Sizeable groups of people identify with Judaism (2 percent), Buddhism (1 percent), and Islam (1 percent).[25] Hinduism and Unitarian Universalism each represent the religious affiliation of just below 1 percent of the general population (See figure 1).[26]

The Bible is very important in the United States. Sixty-eight percent of US homes have a Bible, and 36 percent of people in the United States read the Bible at least weekly.[27] A majority (55 percent) believe that the Bible is the word of God. Thirty percent believe the Bible is the "inspired word of God and has no errors," with some symbolism, and 22 percent believe the Bible is the "actual word of God and should be taken literally, word for word."[28] The Bible is frequently cited in religious debates around sexual and reproductive justice, especially those involving contraception, abortion, and non-marital and same-sex sexual relationships. (See pages 27–28 for more information on the Bible and sexuality issues.)

Religious attendance and affiliation vary by region of the country. Religion is especially important in

Figure 1. US Religious Affiliation

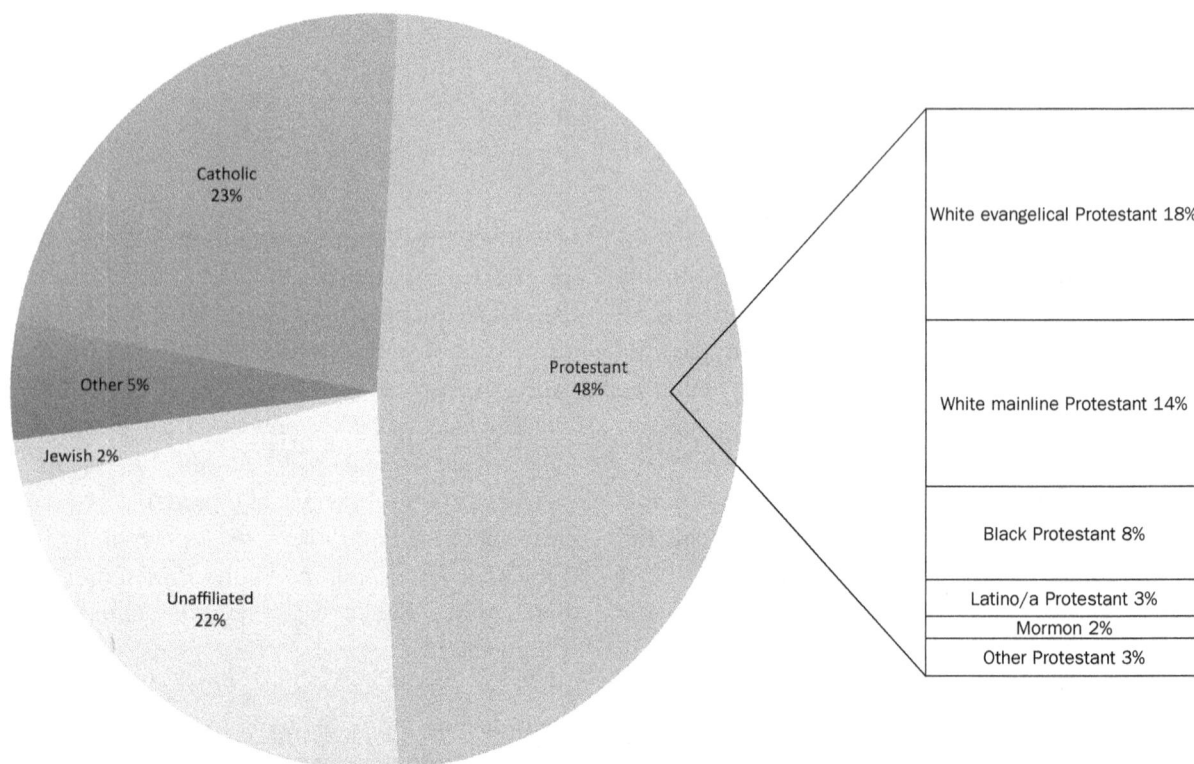

Source: Public Religion Research Institute, American Values Atlas, 2014.[29]

the South. Southerners claim a religious affiliation at a rate (82 percent) 4 percent higher than the national average (78 percent).[30] Southerners as a whole are above the national average in their perception of the importance of religion, their worship attendance, their belief in God, and their frequency of prayer.[31] Sixty-six percent of Southerners say that religion is very important in their lives (compared to 56 percent nationally), 46 percent attend worship weekly (compared to 39 percent nationally), and 66 percent pray daily (compared to 58 percent nationally).[32] Nine of the ten most religious US states are in the South based on the number of adults who report that religion is an important part of their life and that they attend religious services every week or almost every week.[33] Southerners are also more likely to read the Bible.[34] Comparatively, people in the Northeastern states and those in the West are the least religious.

CHANGES IN THE US RELIGIOUS LANDSCAPE

In recent decades, the religious landscape in the United States has been changing. Protestant denominations have been declining, attachment to specific denominational identities has been lessening, and more people have been moving between Protestant denominations than in the past. Nondenominational Protestantism has grown tremendously.

The decline of membership in mainline Protestant denominations is one of the most significant recent changes in religion in the United States. In the 1970s and 1980s, Protestants accounted for about two-thirds of the US population, but beginning in the 1990s, the numbers of US Protestants began to experience a decline (see table 2 and figure 2).[35] Today, Protestants account for slightly less than half

Table 2. Religious Affiliation through the Decades

Year range	1972–82	1983–87	1988–91	1993–98	2000–10	2012–14
Protestant	64.3	63.0	62.8	58.8	55.1	49.5
Catholic	25.1	26.0	25.2	24.6	25.5	25.5
Jewish	2.4	2.1	1.9	2.1	2.0	1.7
None	6.9	7.1	7.6	11.3	16.4	22.0
Other	1.3	1.8	2.5	3.2	1.1	1.3
Total	100	100	100	100	100.1	100

Source: Data compiled from General Social Survey, Cumulative Codebook.[36]

of the US population.[37] The proportion of mainline Protestants has declined from 18.1 percent of the US population in 2007 to 14.7 percent in 2014.[38] Evangelical Protestantism has also experienced a slight decline from 26.3 percent in 2007 to 25.4 percent in 2014.[39] In contrast, the proportion of the general population that identifies as Jewish and Catholic has remained fairly stable during the past five decades.[40]

The Pew Research Center reports that large numbers of people in the United States change religious affiliation during their life. Pew writes that "understanding patterns of religious switching is central to making sense of the trends observed in American religion."[41] When evangelical, mainline, and historically black Protestantism are considered as distinct religious affiliations, as many as four in ten (42 percent) people in the United States have switched religions.[42]

Latino/a communities now compose a larger portion of US churches than ever before. While there has been an overall decline in mainline Protestantism

Figure 2. Trends in Religious Affiliation

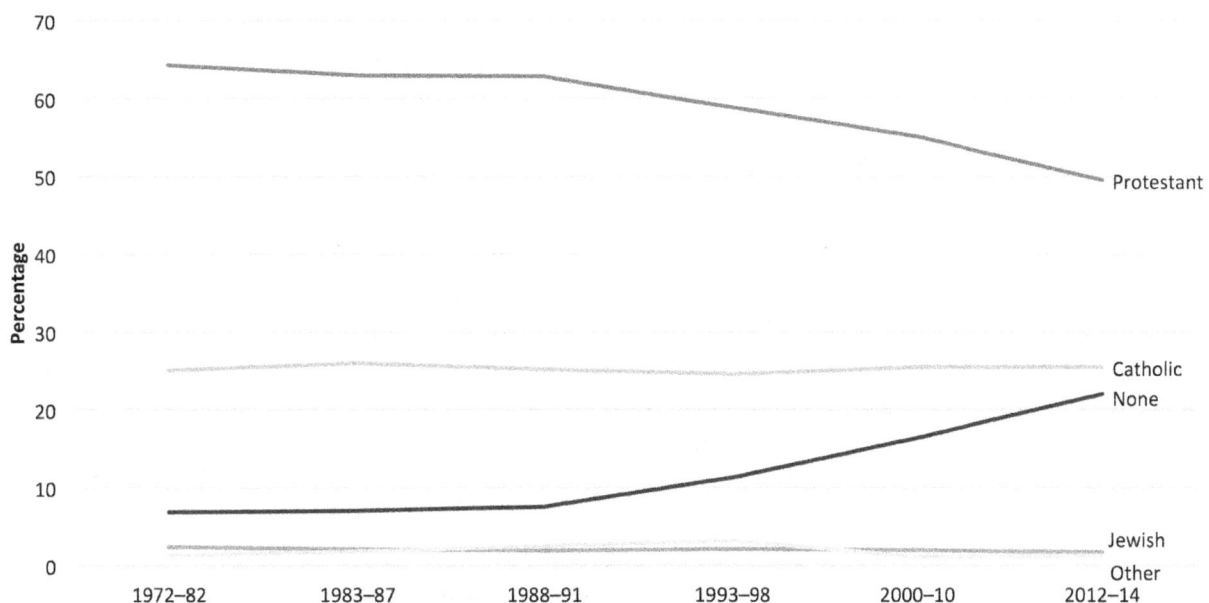

Source: Data compiled from General Social Survey, Cumulative Codebook.[43]

and in the numbers of white Protestants, there has been an increase in the proportion of Latino/a Protestants, especially in the last fifteen years.[44] There has also been a dramatic increase in the proportion of Latino/a Catholics in the last fifteen years.[45] This increase in the proportion of religious Latinos is due to increased migration into the United States and lower rates of disaffiliation and switching religions.

Another important shift in the composition of US religion has been the steady increase of people who identify as atheist or agnostic or claim no religious affiliation in particular. This unaffiliated group, commonly referred to as "nones," has grown from around 7 percent in the 1970s and 1980s to more than 20 percent in the 2010s (see table 2 and figure 2).[46] In 2012, 32 percent of those ages 18–29 were religiously unaffiliated.[47]

However, it is important to understand that this lack of affiliation does not necessarily translate to a lack of religious beliefs or practices. In fact, as a 2008 Pew Research Center report notes, "a large portion (41 percent) of the unaffiliated population says religion is at least somewhat important in their lives, seven in ten say they believe in God and more than a quarter (27 percent) say they attend religious services at least a few times a year."[48] The growing numbers of unaffiliated people in the United States may be altering the character of US religious denominations, but this growth does not necessarily indicate a waning influence of faith in the United States.

PEOPLE OF FAITH SUPPORT AND USE FAMILY PLANNING AND ABORTION SERVICES

Religious affiliation helps shape US perspectives on sexuality, reproduction, contraception, abortion, and LGBTQ issues. Contrary to popular belief, people across religious traditions express support for sexual justice. A majority of the US population supports sexuality education, contraception, and legal access to abortion.

People of all religious backgrounds support comprehensive sexuality education. A 2004 study found that 90 percent of the general public thought sex education was either very important (69 percent) or somewhat important (21 percent) as part of school curricula.[49] A 2011 report by the Public Religion Research Institute (PRRI) found "nearly 8-in-10 (78 percent) Americans favor comprehensive sex education in public schools" and 88 percent of millennials do.[50] In one study, 80 percent of those who self-identified as conservative Christians supported sexuality education in high school and 69 percent of them supported it in junior high/middle school."[51]

Support for contraception is even higher. A 2012 study by PRRI concluded that 87 percent of people in the United States believe that "using artificial birth control methods or contraceptives" is morally acceptable.[52] A similar study by the Pew Research Center in 2012 found that 85 percent of the US population considers "using contraceptives" to be morally acceptable or not a moral issue.[53]

Almost all US women, regardless of religious affiliation, use contraception. A 2011 report from the Guttmacher Institute found that "among women who have had sex, 99 percent have ever used a contraceptive method other than natural family planning (NFP)."[54] Almost all women of faith use contraceptive methods, including Catholic women (87 percent), mainline Protestants (90 percent), and evangelical Protestants (90 percent).[55] Evangelical women are slightly more likely to use the most effective methods. (See figure 3.)

In contrast, views about abortion vary significantly by religious affiliation. When asked about their views on the legality of abortion by PRRI in 2014, a majority of the US population (55 percent) said they believed that abortion should be legal in all or most cases.[56] A majority of people in every region of the country, including the South and the Midwest, hold this opinion. In a different polling question that allowed people to indicate their views on the legality of abortion and its morality, seven in ten said they believed that abortion should be legal or that the government shouldn't prevent a woman from making that decision for herself.[57] A 2014

Figure 3. Contraceptive Use by Faith Tradition

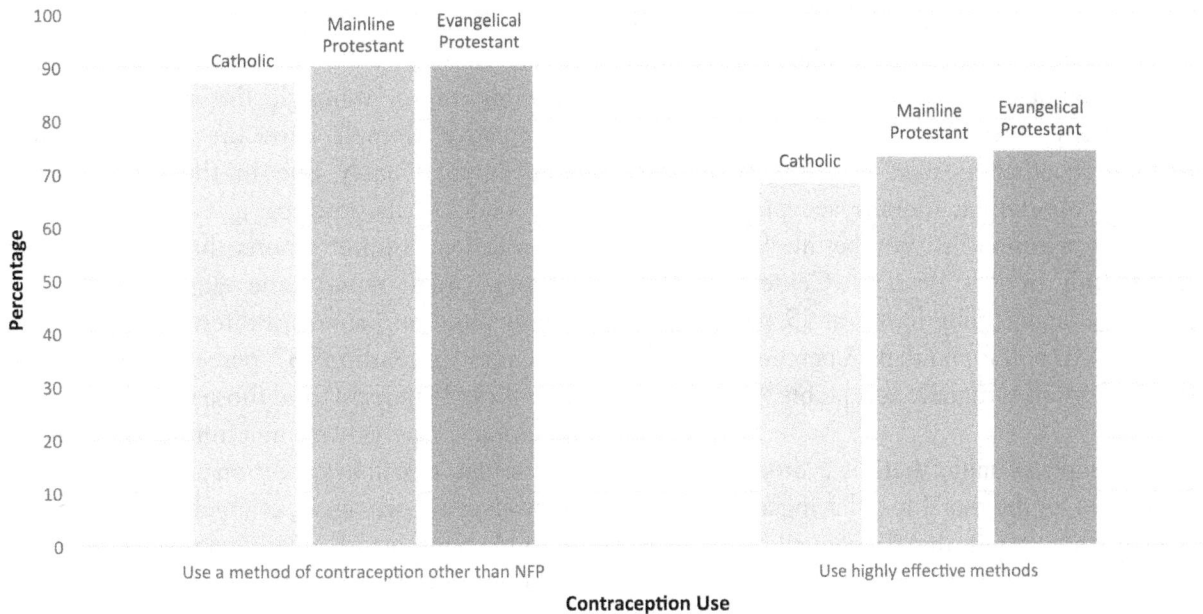

Source: Guttmacher Institute, 2011.[58]

survey found that 57 percent of the US population said at least some health-care professionals in their community should provide legal abortions.[59]

Majorities of most religious groups—with the exception of white evangelical Protestants—believe that abortion should be legal in all or most cases.[60] Eighty-nine percent of Jews,[61] three-quarters (75 percent) of religiously unaffiliated US adults, approximately two-thirds (65 percent) of white mainline Protestants, more than half (56 percent) of black Protestants, and a majority of white (54 percent) and Latino (52 percent) Catholics believe that abortion should be legal in all or most cases.[62] According to the National Latina Institute for Reproductive Health, 74 percent of Latino/a registered voters "agree that a woman has a right to make her own personal, private decisions about abortion without politicians interfering."[63] Nearly one-third (30 percent) of white evangelicals believe abortion should be legal in all or most cases (See table 3).[64]

People in the United States are much more divided about whether having an abortion is "morally acceptable." Studies examining the morality of abortion vary in their conclusions. About half of

Table 3. Views on the Legality of Abortion

	Should be legal in all or most cases (%)	Should be illegal in all or most cases (%)	Don't know (%)
Jews	89	9	2
Unaffiliated	75	20	5
White mainline Protestants	65	30	5
Black Protestants	56	39	5
Latino Catholics	52	42	6
White Catholics	54	42	4
White evangelicals	30	66	3

Source: Pew Research Center, 2013, 2014.[65]

the US population (between 45 percent and 54 percent depending on the study and the wording of the question) believe that having an abortion is morally wrong.[66] These studies differ significantly on the percentage of people who consider abortion to be morally acceptable. While a 2014 study by PRRI reported that one-third (33 percent)[67] believe having an abortion is morally acceptable and a 2012 study reported that number at 39 percent,[68] a 2013 study by Pew Research Center puts that percentage significantly lower, at 15 percent.[69] A 2014 NARAL poll found that 23 percent of people believe abortion is morally acceptable.[70]

Among people of faith, there is a broad range of perspectives on the morality of having an abortion. A recent study reports that 73 percent of Jews and 54 percent of the religiously unaffiliated believe having an abortion is morally acceptable. Among white mainline Protestants, that number drops to four in ten (41 percent). Among white Catholics, 33 percent view having an abortion to be morally acceptable.[71] Only one in four (26 percent) black Protestants believe having an abortion is morally acceptable.[72] That number decreases even further among white evangelicals (13 percent) and Latino/a

Catholics (12 percent). See figure 4 for greater detail.[73]

People from all different religious backgrounds have abortions, although the most religiously conservative women have the lowest abortion rates. Approximately one in three US women have had an abortion by age forty-five.[74] The Guttmacher Institute reports that 73 percent of abortion patients report some religious affiliation.[75] Among abortion patients, Protestants account for the largest proportion (37 percent), followed by Catholics (28 percent) and those with no religious affiliation (27 percent). The Guttmacher Institute reports that "one in five abortion patients identified themselves as born-again, evangelical, charismatic or fundamentalist."[76] When compared with the overall abortion rate in the United States (19.6 abortions per 1,000 women), those who were "born-again, evangelical, or fundamentalist" were least likely to have an abortion (11.4 per 1,000). Protestant women also fell below the overall rate at 15.3 abortions per 1,000 women.[77] In contrast, Catholics (22.3) and the religiously unaffiliated (32.2) had abortions at rates above the overall average (See table 4).[78]

Figure 4. Views on Morality of Abortion by Religious Affiliation

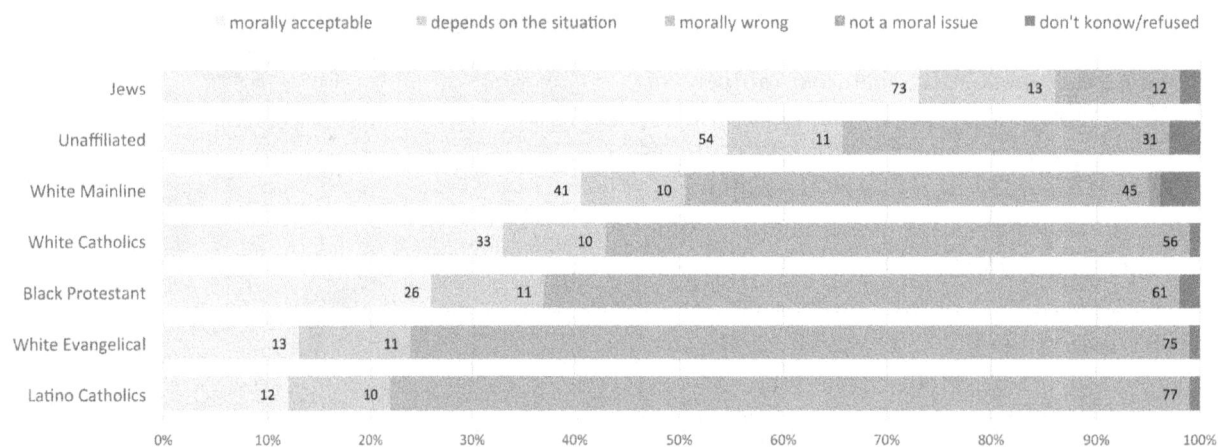

Source: PRRI, LGBT Issues & Trends Survey, 2014.[79]

Table 4. Abortion Rates by Religion

	Rate per 1,000 women
National average	19.6
Born again, charismatic, evangelical, or fundamentalist	11.4
Protestant (overall)	15.4
Roman Catholic	22.3
Religiously unaffiliated	32.2

Source: Obstetrics & Gynecology, 2011. Data are from 2008.[80]

Attitudes about Abortion and Voting Behaviors

People of faith in the United States differ widely in their opinions on the importance of abortion as a public policy issue and in how those opinions affect their voting behavior. Public opinion depends on how the question is posed. When asked if abortion is "a critical issue facing the country," one of many issues, or not that important of an issue, only 18 percent of the general population said abortion is critical,[81] but when asked if abortion is a critical issue to them personally, 31 percent answered in the affirmative.[82] White evangelical Protestants are much more likely to believe abortion is personally critical than white mainline Protestants (45 percent[83] versus 21 percent,[84] respectively), and white evangelical Protestants—some of the staunchest opponents to abortion—are much more mobilized around abortion than white mainline Protestants, Catholics, or the US population as a whole.

Evangelical Protestant fervor around the issue of abortion directly affects their voting practices.[85] In a survey about voter attitudes preceding the 2014 congressional elections, significantly larger percentages of white evangelical Protestants (61 percent) considered abortion a "very important" election issue compared with white mainline Protestants (33 percent), Catholics (48 percent), black Protestants (46 percent), or the general population (46 percent).[86] On the whole, evangelical Protestants consider abortion to be a critical issue and take it into particular consideration when voting. Religiously unaffiliated people, who are more likely to support abortion, are less likely to vote at all.

Morality/Legality Divide

Many more people in the United States think abortion should be legal than believe abortion is morally acceptable. The sexual and reproductive health and justice movement must engage this

Figure 5. Morality/Legality Divide

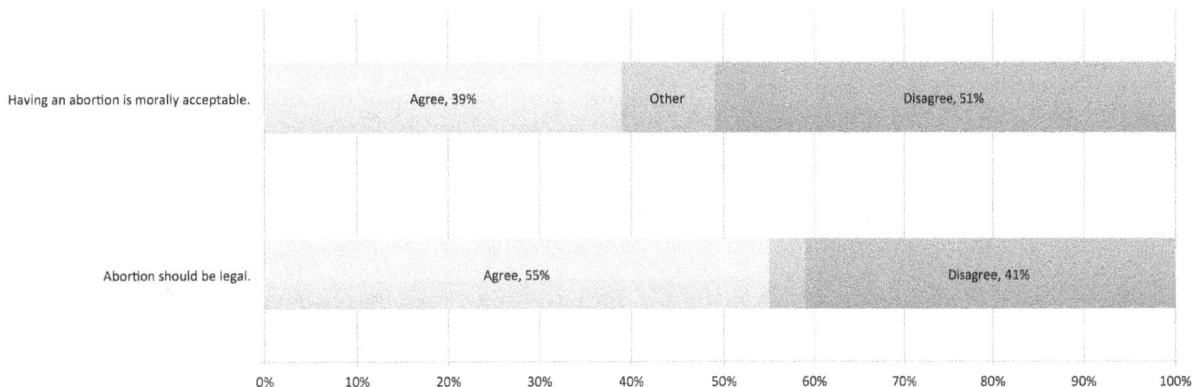

Source: PRRI American Values Atlas, 2014 LGBT Issues & Trends Survey.[87]

"morality/legality divide" in public support. One study found that while 55 percent of the general population thinks abortion should be legal in all or most cases,[88] only 33 percent believe that abortion is morally acceptable (see figure 5).[89] A 2014 NARAL poll found that nearly half (45.5 percent) of US residents agree with the statement, "I am personally against abortion for myself and my family, but I don't believe government should prevent a woman from making that decision for herself."[90]

Almost equal percentages of the US population believe that abortion is morally acceptable and should be legal (23.2 percent) as believe that having an abortion is morally wrong and should be illegal (24.7 percent). Seventy-eight percent of African Americans and 60 percent of Latino/a Americans believe they can disagree with their religions' teachings on abortion and still be considered a person of good standing in their faith.[91]

Seventy-six percent of African Americans who attend religious services on a weekly basis agree that "regardless of how I personally feel about abortion, I believe it should remain legal and women should be able to access safe abortion."[92] (Further discussion of how the sexual and reproductive health and justice movement must address the morality/legality divide is found on pages 34–35.)

HISTORY OF FAITH ENGAGEMENT

Protestant and Jewish clergy were centrally involved in the early days of the birth control movement. In the 1920s, Margaret Sanger engaged clergy to support the development of the American Birth Control League (the forerunner of Planned Parenthood Federation of America). Starting as early as 1929, the first religious denominations passed resolutions in support of birth control. In the 1940s, Planned Parenthood formed its first National Clergyman's Advisory Council, which later published a counseling guidebook for Protestant clergy. In 1946, more than 3,000 clergy signed a statement against religious opposition to birth control provisions. Historian Tom Davis writes that by the end of the 1940s, most major Protestant and Jewish bodies had endorsed birth control for women seeking to avoid pregnancy. In the 1950s, clergy successfully protested Roman Catholic hospitals' decisions to restrict birth control services.[93]

Clergy were a driving force in the movement to secure access to legal abortion. In the 1940s and 1950s, Protestant and Jewish clergy often counseled women who needed "therapeutic abortion." In 1963, the Unitarian Universalist Association passed the first denominational policy statement in favor of reforming abortion laws. In 1967, a *New York Times* front page story announced that twenty-one clergy—nineteen ministers and two rabbis—had founded the Clergy Consultation on Abortion, which grew into a national network of 1,400 clergy referring 100,000 women for safe and affordable abortions. In 1970, clergy were instrumental in opening the nation's first abortion clinic in Manhattan. Following the *Roe v. Wade* decision in 1973, clergy formed the Religious Coalition for Abortion Rights, now known as the Religious Coalition for Reproductive Choice.

Clergy were also at the forefront of the movement to establish sexuality education in public schools. In 1964, Rev. William Genne from the National Council of Churches was one of the founders of SIECUS, the Sex Information and Education Council of the United States. In 1968, the National Council of Churches, the Synagogue Council of America, and the United States Catholic Conference jointly released a statement calling on churches and synagogues to become actively involved in sexuality education in congregations and public schools. The Unitarian Universalist Association (UUA) published the groundbreaking About Your Sexuality curriculum for junior high school youth in 1970, the first comprehensive sex education program for youth in congregations. It has since been replaced by the lifespan sexuality education program Our Whole Lives, which was jointly developed by the UUA and the United Church of Christ.[94]

"What really moved us from the back alley to safe and legal abortion was the clergy who could not stand by and witness the carnage continuing on that scale."[95]

—Dr. David Grimes

During these same years, the Vatican reiterated its opposition to contraception and its view that sexual acts should be open to biological procreation. In the 1930 papal encyclical "Casti Connubii" [On Christian Marriage], Pope Pius XI stated that anyone who "deliberately frustrates" the procreative purpose of the conjugal act sins against

Timeline of Early US Faith Engagement

1920s   Margaret Sanger reaches out to Protestant clergy to support the American Birth Control League

1929–30s   First denominational statements in support of birth control

Resolution at Central Conference of American Rabbis, 1929[96]

Resolution at Universalist General Convention, 1929[97]

Lambeth Conference, Resolution 15, Anglican Communion, 1930[98]

Federal Council of Churches Report on Birth Control 1931[99]

Resolution from Women of Reform Judaism on Birth Control Literature, 1935[100]

1943   Planned Parenthood forms National Clergymen's Advisory Council

1946   3,200 clergy sign statement denouncing religious opposition to birth control

1958   New York City clergy protest hospitals' decision to stop offering contraception

1964   Rev. William Genne joins Dr. Mary Calderone as one of the founders of SIECUS

1967   Clergy Consultation Service on Abortion announced on front page of New York Times

1968   National Council of Churches, Synagogue Council of America, and United States Catholic Conference jointly release statement calling on churches and synagogues to become actively involved in sexuality education in congregations and public schools

1970   New York City clergy establish Women's Services, one of the first freestanding legal abortion clinics in the United States

1971   Unitarian Universalist Association publishes About Your Sexuality, first comprehensive sex education program for youth in congregations

1973   Clergy form Religious Coalition for Abortion Rights (now Religious Coalition for Reproductive Choice)

1973   Catholics for A Free Choice formed (now Catholics for Choice)

nature, law, and God.[101] With the development of the birth control pill in the late 1950s and early 1960s and its widespread adoption, Pope John XXIII charged a commission of lay and ordained Catholics to consider the question of artificial contraception in 1963. An overwhelming majority of the commission concluded that the use of artificial birth control was not an intrinsic moral evil. In 1968, Paul VI rejected the commission's majority report and released "Humanae Vitae" [Of Human Life], which reiterated earlier prohibitions on sexual acts not open to biological procreation.[102]

The day after the release of "Humanae Vitae," eighty-seven theologians released a statement opposing it, a statement more than 600 Catholic theologians would come to endorse. By the mid-1960s, the US Catholic Conference's Family Life Bureau was beginning a program to coordinate national anti-abortion activities. In response, in 1965 NARAL formed the New York State Catholic Women for Abortion Repeal, and in 1973 Catholics For a Free Choice was formed as a national organization growing out of the New York–based Catholics for the Elimination of All Restrictive Abortion and Contraception Laws.[103]

In contrast, evangelical Protestant and most political organizations on the right were not opposed to either family planning or abortion during most of the twentieth century. US religious historian Randall Balmer describes evangelicals as "overwhelmingly indifferent" to the subject of abortion "both before and for several years after Roe."[104] The Southern Baptist Convention passed a resolution in 1971 encouraging Southern Baptists to work for legislation that would "allow the possibility of abortion" under certain circumstances.[105]

After the Roe v. Wade decision, the former president of the Southern Baptist Convention released a public statement of approval. Roe v. Wade was not the catalyst that galvanized the leaders of the religious right, Balmer argues; rather, the catalyst was the loss of federal tax exemptions for private, segregated schools.

In 1976, when the Internal Revenue Service rescinded Bob Jones University's tax-exempt status because of its failure to integrate, evangelical leaders were roused to activism. Balmer writes that Rev. Jerry Falwell and conservative fundraiser Paul Weryrich sought to capitalize on this energy, but were "savvy enough to recognize that organizing grassroots evangelicals to defend racial discrimination would be a challenge...they needed a different issue if they wanted to mobilize evangelical voters on a large scale."[106] Amidst late 1970s concerns about the numbers of legal abortions, the two decided to test the issue of abortion. After key wins by anti-abortion candidates in the 1978 election, these evangelical leaders were convinced that opposition to abortion would galvanize the mass base they sought. Balmer argues that "although abortion had emerged as a rallying cry by 1980, the real roots of the religious right lie not [in] the defense of a fetus but in the defense of racial segregation."[107]

Forty years later, religious voices on the right continue to disproportionately influence public policy about abortion and contraception. The United States Conference of Catholic Bishops (USCCB) continues to play a major role in limiting access to contraception and supporting abortion restrictions across the country. As journalist Patricia Miller notes, the bishops have been constructing a "conscience" narrative for more than a decade about health care, insurance, and reproductive health services: that they are "a violation of an individual's religious liberty, or an employer's, to not allow them to decide what health services other people could and couldn't get in an insurance plan." The USCCB first constructed this narrative during the early 2000s by pushing for "conscience measures" that would, in Miller's words, "allow any employer or insurer to refuse to provide services to which they had a religious or 'moral' objection." Since the 1990s, there have been many mergers and acquisitions between Catholic and non-Catholic hospitals and about half of these mergers and acquisitions have resulted in the reduction of reproductive health care services.[108]

In the 2014 US Supreme Court Case *Burwell v. Hobby Lobby Stores, Inc.*, Hobby Lobby and Conestoga Wood, companies owned by an evangelical Christian family and a Mennonite family, respectively, brought suits against the US Department of Health and Human Services' regulation in the Affordable Care Act requiring employers to provide their employees with contraceptive coverage as a basic health service. These companies claimed that this contraception mandate violates employers' religious freedom. According to Americans United for Separation of Church and State, the Supreme Court found that:

> "The law substantially burdened the plaintiff's religion, and even if the government had a compelling interest in ensuring women's access to contraception, the law was not enforced through the least restrictive means. Therefore, according to RFRA [the Religious Freedom Restoration Act], the government could not force closely held for-profit corporations [with religious objections] to provide health care coverage that includes contraception."[109]

Americans United notes that there are several potential problems with this ruling, both in what the Court considered a "substantial burden" and in its failure to limit the application of the Religious Freedom Restoration Act (RFRA) when it causes harm to a third party. "We believe this is a dramatic departure from what religious freedom truly is," Americans United writes. "Religious freedom means that employers have the right to make medical and moral decisions for themselves, but not for their employees."[110]

The Burwell v. Hobby Lobby decision has invigorated new attempts to deny sexual and reproductive rights on the basis of religious freedom. Sixteen states introduced RFRA bills in the year following the decision; Indiana and Arkansas have already signed RFRAs into law and at least six other bills are still in progress as of this writing. Both Indiana's and Arkansas's laws significantly expand RFRA's coverage, as Americans United describes, "to cases between two private parties,

completely undermining [the original, federal] RFRA's intent to safeguard against governmental intrusion on individual's religious expression."[111]

Mainstream and progressive religious leaders have worked to respond to these recent attacks on sexual and reproductive justice. For example, in 2012, Protestant, Jewish, and Unitarian Universalist denominations supported the White House including contraceptive coverage in health-care reform. More than one thousand religious leaders endorsed the Religious Institute's "Open Letter to Religious Leaders on Family Planning."[112] (See pages 57–58.) More than twenty-five national, faith-related organizations signed on as amicus curiae to a faith brief against Hobby Lobby Stores, Inc., and Conestoga Wood Specialties Corporation.[113] And more than 11,000 people of faith signed on to a petition to "Stand with the Nuns" for contraceptive inclusion.

There are numerous challenges to sexual and reproductive health and justice ahead that intersect directly with religious issues and demand both secular and faith-informed responses. The aftermath of the *Hobby Lobby* decision and the proliferation of state RFRAs demonstrate the need for mainline and progressive religious leaders to reclaim "religious freedom." The public debates about these state RFRAs have focused mostly on LGBTQ issues, specifically the legality of wedding providers (e.g., caterers, photographers, bakers, etc.) denying services to same-sex couples, while the impact of these expanded religious freedom arguments on reproductive health and justice have been largely ignored by the media. RFRA-type laws are being used by medical care providers and pharmacists to deny individuals reproductive health care.[114] These so-called religious freedom laws are actually religious discrimination laws. Many agree with the analysis of Americans United: "Religious freedom means the right to practice your religious beliefs without government interference to the extent that those beliefs do not override the rights of others."[115]

There is also a renewed opportunity to integrate issues related to sexual and reproductive health, rights, and justice into movements for racial and economic equality. During the Civil Rights Movement of the 1950s and '60s, many women's groups worked extensively to ensure that the needs of women of color were integral to the movement's call for justice. The reproductive justice movement, led by organizations of women of color, is taking the lead in articulating why it is essential to address larger social and economic issues facing low-income women and the importance of viewing individual decision making in the larger context of power, privilege, and oppression. The Moral Mondays movement, begun in North Carolina and spreading throughout the United States, has demonstrated how progressive people of faith can be mobilized in broad and consistent coalitions across different issues, including sexual and reproductive health and justice. The Black Lives Matter movement is highlighting the need to urgently address a broad range of issues that address racism, including economic justice, educational inequality, police and prison reform, housing, employment, and the multiple needs of low-income mothers and their children. Reproductive justice advocates and religious leaders are playing central roles in these justice movements. There is new opportunity for collaboration and articulating economic, racial, reproductive, and sexual justice as intersecting social justice issues that carry the same broader goals.

THEOLOGICAL GROUNDING

There are many strong public health arguments for supporting sexual and reproductive health services that are well-known to secular sexual and reproductive health and justice organizations. However, there are also ethical and religious foundations for supporting sexuality education, contraception, abortion, and sexual and reproductive justice. For far too long, conservative and Far Right voices have dominated the religious discourse surrounding these issues. Yet faith-based arguments *against* sexual justice must be countered by voices of faith speaking *for* sexual justice. Far Right religious arguments against LGBTQ rights, comprehensive sexuality education, and access to family planning and abortion services are best countered with clearly articulated faith statements that are based in mainstream and progressive religious values.

People of faith must learn to speak about sexuality issues. Likewise, secular sexual and reproductive health and justice leaders must learn to talk about ethics and values. One participant in the National Colloquium on Faith and Sexual and Reproductive Health and Justice mentioned that many leaders of SRH and RJ organizations feel that they do not speak "faith" and that there is concern that their staff members cannot address these issues because they do not have religious backgrounds or expertise. Several colloquium participants expressed caution that most advocates for sexual and reproductive health and justice lack understanding about religion, and that faith needs to be understood as a "cultural competency" deserving time and training in the same way that race and ethnicity do.

Sexual and reproductive health and justice leaders can learn to use values-based language to support their advocacy work. This does not mean that they need to learn to debate Scripture; rather, they should be able to articulate the values that support sexual and reproductive health and justice. For persons committed to sexual and reproductive justice, offering an effective voice means using both issue-based language and values-based language — theologically informed, scientifically grounded perspectives that reflect an understanding that people of faith embrace sexuality and sexual and reproductive health and justice.

During the past fourteen years, the Religious Institute has developed a series of *Open Letters to Religious Leaders*, multifaith theological statements on sexuality issues. These *Open Letters* are developed at colloquia of theologians, clergy, and activists who articulate the underlying values grounded in religious traditions. The Religious Institute's *Open Letters* provide people of faith and secular SRH and RJ leaders with theologically sound ways to talk about the values of moral agency, respect for life, religious pluralism, integrity in education, and truth-telling. Each of the *Open Letters* has at its foundation the belief that sexuality is a gift to be celebrated rather than a problem to be addressed.

VALUES-BASED LANGUAGE

The following section includes values-based language for many key sexual and reproductive health and justice issues, derived from the Religious Institute's *Open Letters* (see page 55–58).

Sexuality Is a Blessing

Almost all US religions understand sexuality as a divinely bestowed capacity for expressing love and generating life, for mutual companionship, and for pleasure. They teach that sexuality calls for responsibility, respect, and self-discipline; they honor loving, ethical relationships. They understand that sexuality may be celebrated with holiness and integrity, but that it is also vulnerable to exploitation and abuse. Many religious denominations and movements acknowledge that sexual and gender diversity is a blessing.

From these common understandings, however, religious teachings widely diverge. Some faith communities in the United States affirm sexuality as a blessing and have a commitment to sexual health, education, and justice. Others have a deep commitment to some aspects of sexual health, including HIV and teen pregnancy prevention, but remain conflicted on how and whether to include LGBTQ people fully into congregational life. Still others teach that sexuality is to be tightly controlled and restricted to specific acts and relationships.

Sexuality Education with Integrity

Religious traditions value truthful and comprehensive education, including education about sexuality. Beginning at puberty, individuals must have access to comprehensive lifespan sexuality education. Young people need guidance in developing a freely informed conscience and a capacity for moral discernment through sexuality education. Education that respects and empowers young people has more integrity than education based on incomplete information, fear, and shame. Programs that teach abstinence exclusively and withhold information about pregnancy and sexually transmitted infection prevention fail young people.

A commitment to telling the truth calls for full and honest education about sexual and reproductive health. Young people require knowledge and information to develop skills to make ethical and healthy decisions about relationships for themselves in the present and in their future adult lives. It is with guidance and comprehensive information and education about sexuality—education that includes abstinence, contraception, and STI prevention—that young people will be able to make responsible decisions.

Respect for Life

Religious traditions affirm that life is sacred. They celebrate the divinely bestowed blessings of generating life and assuring that life can be sustained and nurtured. Religious traditions have different beliefs about the value of fetal life, often according greater value as fetal development progresses. Science, medicine, law, and philosophy contribute to this understanding. The teaching of many traditions is that the health and life of the person carrying the fetus must take precedence over the life of the fetus.

The sanctity of human life is best upheld when it is created intentionally and when pregnancies and childbirths are healthy and safe. It is precisely because life and parenthood are so precious that no individual should be forced to carry a pregnancy to term. Families in all of their diverse forms are best upheld in environments where there is love and respect, children thrive, and all are protected. It is unacceptable for society to impose limits on family size or to discriminate against those who do not choose to be parents.

Abortion Is Morally Acceptable

Decisions about abortion and reproductive health are serious moral decisions. Women are moral agents with the right and responsibility to make their own decisions about procreation, whether or not to have children, the size of their family, spacing of children, and whether or not an abortion is justified in their specific circumstances. Such decisions are best made when they are informed by conscience, serious reflection, insights from one's faith and values, and consultation with a caring partner, family members, and spiritual counselor, if appropriate. The moral agency of women must be upheld. "A just society does not compel individuals to continue an undesired pregnancy."[116]

Biblical Texts

Biblical texts are silent on modern contraception, and they neither condemn nor prohibit abortion. They do, however, call us to act compassionately and justly when facing difficult moral decisions. Scriptural stories honor and welcome diverse families, the care of children, and moral and just decision making. The scriptural mandate to care for the most marginalized and the most vulnerable calls us to assure access to contraception, abortion, and comprehensive sexuality education for all people. A religious commitment to social and economic justice requires a commitment to sexual and reproductive justice.

MORAL IMPERATIVE TO ACCESS TO FAMILY PLANNING AND ABORTION SERVICES

Religions have a venerable tradition supporting healing, health care, disease prevention, and health promotion. They also express commitment to the most marginalized, the most vulnerable, and those most likely to be excluded. In a just world, all people would have equal access to contraception

---

NATIONAL RELIGIOUS LEADERS SUPPORT CONTRACEPTIVE ACCESS

The following Religious Institute statement, released March 18, 2014, was endorsed by forty-five national religious leaders, including current and former presidents of denominations, leaders of multifaith organizations, and presidents and deans of seminaries. It is an example of using theological statements to support reproductive health services.

"As religious leaders, we support universal access to contraception. We believe that all persons should be free to make personal decisions about their reproductive lives, their health, and the health of their families that are informed by their culture, faith tradition, religious beliefs, conscience, and community. We affirm, in accordance with each of our faith traditions, that ensuring equal access to contraceptives through insurance coverage is a moral good. Including contraceptives as a covered service does not require anyone to use it; excluding contraceptive coverage for those who choose to plan and space their families with modern methods of birth control will effectively translate into coercive childbearing for many.

We support social justice. We recognize the dignity and worth of each and every member of our communities—including those uniquely vulnerable to the effects of unequal access to health care due to race, class, sex, sexual orientation, gender identity, disability, or geography.

We support religious freedom. Religious freedom means that each individual has the right to exercise their own beliefs and the right not to have others' beliefs forced upon them. We believe no employer has the right to deny women who work for them basic health care. Individuals must have the right to accept or reject the principles of their own faith without legal restrictions.

No single religious voice can speak for all faith traditions on contraception, nor should government take sides on religious differences. We call on our government to respect the beliefs and values of everyone's faith by safeguarding equal access to contraception for those whose conscience leads them to use it."[117]

---

and abortion services. The denial of these services effectively translates into coercive childbearing and is an insult to human dignity. Current measures that limit access to contraception and abortion services are punitive and do nothing to promote moral decision making. When there is a conflict between the conscience of the provider and the person receiving care, the institution delivering the services has an obligation to assure that the person's conscience and decisions will be respected and that access to reproductive health care will be provided either directly or through referral.

COUNTERING OPRESSION

The lack of sexual and reproductive health services in the United States is an affront to moral agency and a threat to justice and equality. For individuals and families to thrive, they must be free from oppression. Commitment to sexual and reproductive justice demands work to ameliorate poverty, social inequities, ignorance, sexism, ageism, environmental degradation, racism, unjust immigration policies, and violence in all

of its forms, including intimate partner violence, which may render an individual virtually powerless to choose freely. There must also be a societal commitment to full and equal educational and employment opportunities for women and girls.

RELIGIOUS PLURALISM

No government committed to human rights and democracy can privilege the teachings of one religion over another or deny individuals their religious freedom. Individuals must have the right to accept or reject the principles of their own faith without legal restrictions. No single religious voice can speak for all faith traditions on abortion, contraception, sexuality education, or other topics related to sexual and reproductive justice. The government should not take sides on religious differences by making specific religious doctrine on these issues the law of the United States. Religious groups themselves must respect the beliefs and values of other faiths, since no single faith can claim final moral authority in public discourse.

OPEN LETTERS TO RELIGIOUS LEADERS ON SEXUALITY ISSUES

- Religious Declaration on Sexual Morality, Justice, and Healing

- Open Letter to Religious Leaders about Sex Education

- Open Letter to Religious Leaders on Marriage Equality

- Open Letter to Religious Leaders on Abortion as a Moral Decision

- Open Letter to Religious Leaders on Adolescent Sexuality

- Open Letter to Religious Leaders on Sexual and Gender Diversity

- Open Letter to Religious Leaders on Assisted Reproductive Technologies

- Open Letter to Religious Leaders on Maternal Mortality and Reproductive Justice

- Open Letter to Religious Leaders on Family Planning

All Open Letters can be found at www.religiousinstitute.org/endorse

ENGAGING FAITH IN SEXUAL AND REPRODUCTIVE HEALTH, RIGHTS, AND JUSTICE

The Religious Institute conducted four surveys in preparing this white paper, with four different groups: the largest and most influential national sexual and reproductive health and justice organizations; denominations and denominational groups that work on reproductive health advocacy; national organizations that focus on the intersection of religion with sexual and reproductive health, rights, and justice; and foundations that provide support for sexual and reproductive health, rights, and justice. A total of forty-five organizations completed surveys.

SECULAR ORGANIZATIONS

In the early history of the sexual and reproductive health movement, religious leaders were central to efforts to defend access to contraception and establish abortion rights. However, during the past thirty-five years, most secular organizations whose work focuses on sexual and reproductive health, rights, and justice have done less to engage religious leaders and people of faith, and few effectively articulate a moral vision for their work. Yet advocates who work for sexual and reproductive health and justice organizations, whether they are personally religious or not, are motivated by the same values that inspire people of faith: a passion for justice, a desire to ensure health and well-being for all, and a call to protect individual dignity and self-worth.

In February 2015, the Religious Institute conducted an online study of major national sexual and reproductive health and justice organizations to understand the extent of their faith commitments (the six national organizations within this field that have an explicit focus on religion were surveyed separately, and are discussed on pages 42–44). The study focused on these secular organizations' work at the intersection of religion with sexual and reproductive health and justice, inquiring about current work to engage religious leaders and people of faith, interest in engaging religion, attitudes about religion, and previous engagement with faith-based SRH and RJ organizations. The study had a 91 percent response rate; nineteen organizations participated (for the full list of participating organizations, see page 60).

The results indicated that few of the national secular SRH and RJ organizations are proactively engaging religion in their work. Most (between 72–89 percent depending on the specific issue) have not published materials that address faith. Two-thirds (68 percent) do not involve faith leaders in their organization's public policy efforts. Only one-third (32 percent) reported doing outreach to people of faith, and just a quarter (26 percent) reported outreach to faith leaders (see figure 6).

Among the organization leaders who responded, only Advocates for Youth and Planned Parenthood Federation of America have faith-based projects. Planned Parenthood Federation of America has had some form of a clergy advisory board since the 1940s. Advocates for Youth explicitly discusses the importance of faith on its website:

> "Advocates for Youth joins with millions of religious and spiritual youth and adults in believing that faith, and a positive approach to healthy sexuality, are not mutually exclusive. Some religious communities promote unhealthy or discriminatory ideology that

damages public health. But religious communities also serve as centers of support, resistance, and political action."[118]

In 2008, Advocates for Youth created the Muslim Youth Project to "meet the reproductive and sexual health needs of Muslim-identified youth." The program is designed to "determine the most effective ways to reach out and serve young Muslims" and to help Muslim youth become "leaders in their own communities on the issues of sexual and reproductive health and justice."[119]

Many of the surveyed organizations say they are working to respond to negative faith-based attacks on sexual and reproductive rights. Sixty-three percent of the organizations reported doing work to counter conscience/refusal clauses or RFRA-based arguments. The ACLU Reproductive Health Program, the National Women's Law Center, and the Center for Reproductive Rights have well-developed legal efforts to respond to Far Right religious attacks. For example, the ACLU's website says, "The ACLU works to ensure that women are

not denied information and the health care they need because of the religious views of their health care providers…. Religion is being used as an excuse to discriminate against and harm others."[120]

Only a few of the surveyed SRH and RJ organizations have allocated resources or made structural commitments to work on religion in the context of their larger work. For most, their strategic plans, mission statements, and programs do not address religious leaders or people of faith. Nearly nine out of ten (89 percent) have no mention of religion or religious leaders in their strategic plan. Seventy-nine percent of the organizations have no religious leader on their Board of Directors. Eight out of ten (79 percent) have no staff with responsibility for religion. None of the organizations surveyed reported that more than 10 percent of their annual budget goes to addressing religion, and the majority (53 percent) reported that their organization allocates no resources to addressing religion.

On the other hand, almost all (89 percent) of the surveyed organizations have worked with at least

Figure 6. Work of SRH and RJ Organizations on Faith

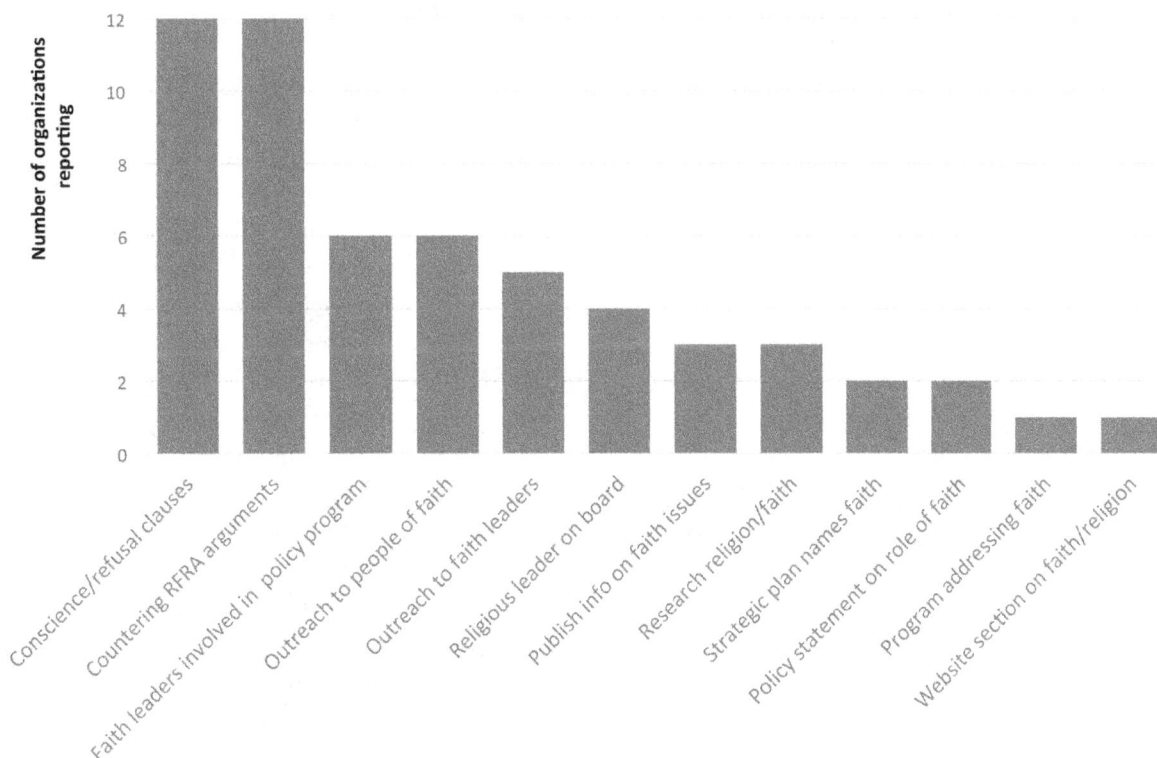

one faith-based sexual and reproductive health and justice organization (e.g., the Religious Institute, the Religious Coalition for Reproductive Choice, Catholics for Choice, and the National Council of Jewish Women) during the past five years. The executives at three out of four of the organizations (74 percent) regularly read materials published by these organizations. More than half (53 percent) have asked for faith-based organizations' assistance in obtaining support from faith leaders for their work. More than a third (37 percent) have requested help in obtaining a religious presence at hearings, rallies, or lobby days; articles on faith support (for blogs, newsletters, etc.); and suggestions for media spokespeople on religion and reproductive rights. The vast majority of the respondents (84 percent) agreed that it was important for the SRH and RJ movements to engage people of faith and religious leaders in advocacy efforts, and three out of four (74 percent) said that they are interested in engaging faith leaders and people of faith more widely in their work.

The organization leaders also expressed nuanced perspectives on the role religion has played in debates about reproductive rights in the United States. On the one hand, nearly eight in ten (79 percent) agreed that "religious leaders have hurt reproductive rights in the United States." However, the same percentage (79 percent) agreed that "religious leaders have helped secure reproductive rights in the United States." When asked if they thought religion has done more to hurt or more to help, 63 percent agreed that "religion has done more to hurt reproductive rights than secure them in the United States."

Nevertheless, this caution about religion does not deter their interest in more fully engaging religion in the SRH and RJ movement or decrease their belief in the importance of faith. When asked if they agreed with the statement "I think it is important for the sexual and reproductive health and justice field to do more to engage mainstream and progressive people of faith and religious leaders in our advocacy efforts," every respondent agreed or strongly agreed. One respondent affirmed both

the importance of religion in the movement and the need for resources, saying that engaging faith in the movement is both "very important" and "under-resourced." Another respondent pointed to the role religious leaders could play in developing values-based language around SRH and RJ issues, describing how religious leaders could "speak to the moral dimensions of allowing women agency in making choices about their reproductive health and lives." Many respondents also pointed to the fact that religious voices can show that "there are religious viewpoints on both sides" of the issues.

"We need faith leaders to model faith-based supportive views on reproductive justice and specifically abortion. 'I support X because of my faith, not in spite of it.'"

—*Colloquium participant*

When asked what they would need in order to do more work engaging religion, respondents most often said they need funding to do more with religious leaders and people of faith. Forty-two percent said that in order to do more work engaging faith leaders and people of faith, their organization would need "dedicated financial resources." Significant numbers of leaders expressed a need for materials about what faith traditions say about sexual and reproductive health, rights, and justice (37 percent) and religious freedom (32 percent). One in four (26 percent) said their organization needs staff training on faith. Their responses also confirmed the need for staff training and education specific to faith engagement. For example, none of the respondents answered "strongly agree" to a question that asked whether spokespeople for their organization had effectively debated religious leaders on the right, and only two of the nineteen organizations replied "strongly agree" to a question asking if they were knowledgeable about US faith traditions.

Discussion

While most of the surveyed sexual and reproductive health and justice organizations say they are interested in engaging faith and many do limited work, very few have dedicated resources to religious engagement. As a whole, these organizations have not made commitments to addressing religion. Their board composition, budgets, guiding documents, programs, and public policies indicate that faith is at best marginalized in their work. The current work being done to engage faith has been mostly combatting or containing religion's negative reach into social and political issues or periodically bringing a "faith face" to an advocacy issue.

Many religious leaders who have worked with SRH and RJ groups comment that they are more often used for photo opportunities rather than systematic engagement. It is not enough, as Rev. Harry Knox says, "to collar up the conversation." Effective faith/secular partnerships require significant investments in personnel, resources, time, and a sustained commitment by organizational leaders. These partnerships succeed best when secular organizations view religion and faith as a cultural competency and make it part of the professional development of their staffs.

Several participants in the National Colloquium on Faith and Sexual and Reproductive Health and Justice noted that it would be difficult for an employee to be open about their personal involvement in a faith community at many of the national SRH and RJ organizations. Just half of the executives from these organizations responded in the survey that they have a personal religious affiliation, and only a third report that they attend a religious service at least once a month. Especially given the perception among many that religion is hostile to sexual and reproductive health and justice issues, it is important to ensure that workplaces within this field are welcoming environments for people of faith. Indeed, SRH and RJ organizations may find untapped potential for religion work among people of faith within their own organization. Many staff at these organizations also struggle with how to discuss their work with family members who may

oppose it on religious grounds. As one colloquium participant mentioned, "this is a serious human resources issue."

It is important to build on the partnerships between secular SRH and RJ organizations and organizations like the Religious Institute that work at the intersection of faith with sexual and reproductive health and justice. SRH and RJ organizations consistently look to these faith-based organizations for help engaging faith voices. These partnerships are ripe for expansion. Many of the resources secular SRH and RJ organizations expressed that they would need in order to address religion are materials that faith-based SRH and RJ organizations already possess. These organizations are uniquely poised to provide educational information on how faith communities can address sexual and reproductive health and justice issues, as well as religious freedom. Faith-based SRH and RJ organizations can also offer staff cultural competency training on faith, including why discussing morality and values is important and providing information about US faith traditions.

The leadership of faith-based sexual and reproductive health and justice organizations and their faith networks can also be a resource to help secular SRH and RJ organizations create and articulate their own values-based missions and visions. Including religious leaders on the national boards of these organizations can ensure that ethics and values are articulated in the organizations' culture, strategic plan, and resources. SRH and RJ organizations can consider adding the values of compassion, empathy, moral agency, justice, right relations, and other values to their own mission statements and materials. A values-based vision is not a statement of religious belief; rather, it is a statement of the values that provide the foundation for the organization's work. The National Latina Institute for Reproductive Health, for example, has what they call a "core values" statement that reads: "We believe in the principles of salud, dignidad, y justicia (health, dignity, and justice) and work that is community rooted, culturally responsive, and sex positive."[121]

Secular organizations that have not engaged faith-based allies can begin by developing relationships with key religious leaders nationally. These relationships can be helpful in identifying shared concerns and creating collaborative projects, and they can lead to long-term partnerships. Secular advocates for sexual and reproductive health and justice might also consider the vital resources that faith communities can provide at the local level. Religious activists have valuable skills in organizing, communications, and networking. Congregations can provide volunteers, meeting space, grassroots support, and high profile venues for public action.

Sexual and reproductive health and justice organizations need to understand that relationships with religious organizations are intensive to develop. Faith communities are involved with multiple issues. Multifaith advocacy requires equal and broad-ranging partnerships, not single-issue campaigns. They must be based on authentic, non-transactional relationships committed to mutual learning and development. Advocates who seek to engage colleagues from faith traditions in SRH and RJ advocacy must demonstrate that they are willing to support a broader range of justice issues—such as immigration, poverty alleviation, and racial justice—that reflect their colleagues' concerns and those of their congregations.

Sexual and reproductive health and justice organizations must intentionally address the morality/legality divide among the US public. The fact that almost half of people in the United States think abortion is not moral but should be legal in some circumstances reflects both the success of the SRH and RJ movement in presenting the need for abortion to be safe and legal and the success of the anti-abortion movement in presenting abortion in most circumstances as unethical or immoral. "Keep your laws off my body" was an early and often-repeated message, emphasizing legality concerns. An editorial in *The American Prospect* in the fall of 2014 expresses the rights argument this way: "Only by reclaiming abortion as a fundamental right and normal part of health care can the pro-choice movement hope to win in the long run."[122] A recent

cartoon on Tumblr, sponsored by Abortion Looks Like, goes even further in explaining abortion as a medical procedure without moral significance: "I wish having an abortion was treated like going to the dentist."[123]

Whether one personally agrees with these legality-based messages or not, they are unlikely to resonate with the 45 percent of the US population who believe that abortion is morally unacceptable or the vast majority who believe that abortion is a moral issue. A 2013 study reported that "regardless of their views about the legality of abortion, most Americans think that having an abortion is a moral issue."[124] Sixty-four percent of US adults said having an abortion was a matter of morality.[125]

The colloquium participants agreed that there needs to be a positive moral framing of abortion, and such a framework must articulate the importance of abortion as a moral good. Noting that abortion support varies by the reason that is given for having one, participants concurred that there is a need to help people "move from judgment to compassion." As one participant noted, "We need to connect our support for sexual and reproductive health and rights to larger issues and dynamics—compassion, pluralism, respect, justice—not to judgment. Our overall call is bigger than sexual or reproductive health decisions. It's about everyone being able to make decisions according to their own values, and having the resources to do so."

Advocates for Youth's "1 in 3" campaign will have great resonance with religious leaders and communities.[126] The stories that are part of the "1 in 3" campaign will help people understand that the morality of abortion is based in everyday, lived realities. The organizations Faith Aloud and Exhale could be helpful in providing stories that illustrate that abortion is a personal moral decision that can only be made by the individual who is pregnant. The many organizations working on changing the cultural conversation on abortion must engage issues of morality directly in their networks, including involving religious voices at the outset. Stories can also help move the public from judgment to compassion. The public needs to hear stories connected to faith, stories that say, "my faith helped me decide to have an abortion," "my faith leader counseled me to listen to what I knew was right for me and my family," and "my faith sustained me during a difficult time of unplanned pregnancy." There should also be dissemination of stories of reproductive health clinics that use chaplains and stories of faith leaders who have stood up for reproductive justice. Good preachers use stories to illustrate their points, and the availability of stories about people who have had abortions will help religious leaders share their convictions with their congregations.

The sexual and reproductive health and justice movement can acknowledge that abortion is a complex moral decision without stigmatizing those who have abortions. The movement can also speak forcefully against those who would deny abortion services, picket clinics, and pass restrictions that penalize people who are seeking care as acting immorally. Coercing an individual into continuing an unwanted pregnancy is unethical and violates moral agency.

Sexual and reproductive health and justice does not exist in a vacuum—it cannot be effectively addressed as a single issue. Access to sexual and reproductive health care for all cannot be achieved without addressing how different experiences and oppressions intersect. Many faith leaders will resonate with calls for reproductive justice, and a larger concern for marginalized and vulnerable communities. Faith communities are more likely to mobilize around SRH and RJ issues—and their efforts are more likely to be effective—if they are addressed in a broader social and economic justice framework. Faith leaders who have not yet worked on sexuality issues but are already committed to alleviating poverty are potential new advocates for the SRH and RJ movement. In Southern states, organizations like SisterReach and SisterSong are leading this approach to faith organizing.

Upholding women's moral agency—as well as women's legal rights—must be at the center of

the discussion. A commitment to moral agency and reproductive justice also means, as Marlene Fried says in a recent essay, that the sexual and reproductive health and justice movement must "affirm, with the same passion and commitment it accords to abortion rights, the right of an individual woman to make her own decision to have a child, regardless of her resources or circumstances."[127]

DENOMINATIONS AND RELIGIOUS LEADERS

There is a long history of religious denominations advocating for sexual and reproductive health. Religious leaders have played a significant role in securing the rights and access to abortion and contraception in this country. As early as the 1929 resolutions on birth control by the Central Conference of American Rabbis and the Universalist General Convention and as recently as the Union for Reform Judaism's 2014 statement on *Hobby Lobby*, Jewish movements and Protestant denominations have advocated for securing reproductive health and rights.

Many denominations continue this advocacy today. Seven denominations are official coalition members of the Religious Coalition for Reproductive Choice (RCRC). They are the Episcopal Church (USA), the Jewish Reconstructionist Movement, the United Methodist Church, the Metropolitan Community Church, the Union for Reform Judaism, the Unitarian Universalist Association, and the United Church of Christ. Some denominations have affiliated organizations that support women's health issues and are also members of RCRC. These include Disciples for Choice, the Episcopal Women's Caucus, the Lutheran Women's Caucus, Presbyterians Affirming Reproductive Options, the Unitarian Universalist Women's Federation, Women of Reform Judaism, and the Women's League of Conservative Judaism.

The Religious Institute conducted a survey of religious denominations or their SRH or RJ working group. The survey had an 82 percent response rate with a total of nine completing the survey (for the full list of responding organizations, see page 60). The denominations surveyed only include those that have worked for sexual and reproductive health and justice and excluded denominations which are actively hostile to the goals of the SRH and RJ movement.

Denominations use a variety of terms to refer to their sexual and reproductive health and justice efforts. The most common term used is "reproductive rights." Nine out of ten (89 percent) use this term. A large majority (67 percent) use the frame of "reproductive health." A minority of those surveyed use "reproductive justice" (33 percent) or "pro-choice" (22 percent).

Three out of four (77 percent) of these religious denominations report they are moderately to very active on issues related to sexual and reproductive health and justice. Eighty-nine percent include family planning, abortion, and/or reproductive justice in their public policy work. Among those who said their policy or advocacy work includes SRH and RJ issues, all had signed on to coalition letters, three out of four had top officials who spoke out on these issues, and almost all (88 percent) encourage their congregations to engage in advocacy on these issues.

Eighty-nine percent of the surveyed denominations have worked with faith-based sexual and reproductive health and justice organizations (e.g., Religious Institute, RCRC, Catholics for Choice, the National Council of Jewish Women, etc.) in the past five years. A majority of the denominations have published materials on faith and SRH and RJ issues. Seventy-eight percent have published materials on sexuality education, 58 percent have published materials on LGBTQ issues, 56 percent have published materials on abortion, and half have published materials on family planning.

Most of these denominations have official policies on sexual and reproductive health and justice, often first passed forty to fifty years ago (see "Denominations Support Sexual Justice" box). Eighty-nine percent of the surveyed denominations

have an official policy on sexuality education and a policy on legal abortion. Half of the denominations have a policy on public funding for abortion services. Two-thirds have policies on LGBTQ equality. Sixty-three percent have passed a policy on domestic family planning in the past five years.

Several denominations have continued to release statements on sexual and reproductive health and justice in recent years. The Alliance of Baptists, for example, released a formal statement "on Lifelong Sexual Education, Sexual & Reproductive Rights, and Opposing Sexual Injustice and Violence" in 2012. In 2013, the Unitarian Universalist Association released a statement in commemoration of the anniversary of *Roe v. Wade*.[128] The Metropolitan Community Church and the Fellowship of Affirming Ministries jointly released a similar statement in 2013.[129] In 2014, the Religious Action Center of the Union for Reform Judaism released a statement on the Supreme Court ruling on *Burwell v. Hobby Lobby*. Many denomination leaders have recently endorsed multifaith statements in support of reproductive health and rights. For example, in 2012, sixteen denominational leaders signed a statement on including contraceptive coverage in health care. In 2015, seventeen denominations and their working groups signed a statement against the twenty-week abortion ban (see "Denomination and Denominational Working Groups Opposing Twenty-Week Abortion Ban" box).

Many of these denominational statements offer nuanced framing of sexual and reproductive health and justice issues using morality, values-based, or religious language. Several denominations speak to the moral complexity of abortion. In their 2012 statement on "Responsible Parenthood," the United Methodist Church, for example, states: "We reject simplistic answers to abortion...[those that] regard all abortion as murders, or on the other hand, regard abortions as medical procedures without moral significance."[130] The Unitarian Universalist Association (UUA) also lifts up the "morally complex nature of abortion" in one of its many statements.[131] Many of these denominational statements also lift up the primacy of the individual conscience in making decisions. The UUA also mentions the importance of individual choices, calling for "tolerance and compassion for persons whose choices differ from our own."[132]

Many denominations have explicit policies to explore the tension between those in their memberships who hold differing opinions about abortion. In the words of a 2007 Disciples of Christ policy resolution, "all Christians affirm the sanctity

of life and the dignity of women."[133] The Disciples of Christ has a preferred option for prevention: "proactive prevention seeks to find common ground on the issue of abortion by focusing on the prevention of unwanted pregnancies and by supporting pregnant women rather than focusing on the divisive and polarizing debates between pro-choice and pro-life advocates." The Episcopal Church, in a 1994 resolution, states that special care must be taken to ensure that the "individual

---

DENOMINATIONS SUPPORT SEXUAL JUSTICE

Religious Support for Sexuality Education

The following denominational bodies have passed policies supporting sexuality and/or HIV/AIDS education in public schools:
- American Baptist Church, USA
- Central Conference of American Rabbis
- Church of the Brethren
- The Episcopal Church
- Evangelical Lutheran Church in America
- Jewish Reconstructionist Federation
- Metropolitan Community Churches
- Presbyterian Church (USA)
- Reform Church in America
- Union for Reform Judaism
- Unitarian Universalist Association
- United Church of Christ
- The United Methodist Church
- United Synagogue of Conservative Judaism

Religious Support for Contraception

The following denominational bodies have passed policies in support of family planning:
- Alliance of Baptists
- American Baptist Church, USA
- Central Conference of American Rabbis
- Church of the Brethren
- The Episcopal Church
- Evangelical Lutheran Church in America
- Jewish Reconstructionist Federation

- The Lutheran Church—Missouri Synod
- Mennonite Church USA
- Metropolitan Community Churches
- Presbyterian Church (USA)
- Seventh-day Adventist Church
- Union for Reform Judaism
- Unitarian Universalist Association
- United Church of Christ
- The United Methodist Church
- United Synagogue of Conservative Judaism

Religious Support for Abortion

The following denominational bodies have passed policies in support of legal abortion:
- Alliance of Baptists
- Central Conferences of American Rabbis
- Christian Church (Disciples of Christ)
- The Episcopal Church
- Evangelical Lutheran Church in America
- Jewish Reconstructionist Federation
- Metropolitan Community Churches
- Moravian Church—Northern Province
- Presbyterian Church (USA)
- Society for Humanistic Judaism
- Union for Reform Judaism
- Unitarian Universalist Association
- United Church of Christ
- The United Methodist Church
- United Synagogue of Conservative Judaism

> ### DENOMINATION AND DENOMINATIONAL WORKING GROUPS OPPOSING TWENTY-WEEK ABORTION BAN, 2015
>
> - Central Conference of American Rabbis
> - Disciples for Choice
> - Disciples Justice Action Network
> - Episcopal Women's Caucus
> - Global Justice Institute (Metropolitan Community Churches)
> - Methodist Federation for Social Action
> - Metropolitan Community Church
> - Muslims for Progressive Values
> - Presbyterian Voices for Justice
>
> - Reconstructionist Rabbinical College and Jewish Reconstructionist Communities
> - Society for Humanistic Judaism
> - Union for Reform Judaism
> - Unitarian Universalist Association
> - Unitarian Universalist Women's Federation
> - United Church of Christ, Justice and Witness Ministries
> - Women's League for Conservative Judaism
> - Women of Reform Judaism

conscience is respected."[134] The statement continues by stating that "the responsibility of individuals to make informed decisions in this matter [of abortion] is acknowledged and honored as the position of this Church."[135]

Several denominations have also applied a justice framework for sexual and reproductive health and rights. The United Church of Christ, for example, states succinctly that "abortion is a social justice issue."[136] Both the Metropolitan Community Churches (MCC) and the Unitarian Universalist Association have adopted reproductive justice framing. In a 2013 statement the MCC states:

"We embrace the principles of the reproductive justice movement...[we seek to] eliminate[e] conditions around the world that compromise a woman's right to choose and impede every woman's ability to enjoy lives of social, political, physical, spiritual and economic wellbeing."[137]

The UUA General Assembly voted in 2012 to make reproductive justice a denomination-wide "Congregational Study/Action Issue (CSAI)" for the next four years. The UUA website in discussing the adoption of the CSAI on Reproductive Justice says:

"We advocate not only for the freedom of those choices in each person's life journey, but also for the ability of all families and communities to realize a sense of wholeness with regard to their sexual and reproductive lives. We create safe and healthy environments for children in our faith communities and campaign publicly for just and compassionate laws for family planning, reproductive health, and gender equality."[138]

The CSAI process involved the development of a curriculum for adult religious education on reproductive justice, in-depth resources on reproductive justice, small group reflection sessions, congregational resources (e.g., sermons, worship services, liturgical calendar, etc.), webinars, discussion questions, a DVD, and several background documents. The resulting statement, excerpted on page 39, was adopted at the June 2015 UUA General Assembly at the conclusion of the first three years of study and action.

There is a perception that religious denominations have been less involved in sexual and reproductive health and justice issues than they were in the 1960s and 1970s. Sally Steenland, writing in a

2011 report for the Center for American Progress, explained the lessening of commitment this way:

"Long-standing faith allies—especially in mainline denominations—are facing increased opposition from within and outside their ranks. Allies within the Presbyterian, United Methodist, and Lutheran churches are facing challenges from groups like the Institute on Religion and Democracy and other well-funded forces that have infiltrated church representation in order to repeal denominational policies supporting sexual and reproductive rights. These groups aim to defund church programs that support women's issues, isolate leaders who work on them, and shift the denomination in a far more conservative, even reactionary, direction. In addition, conservative members within the churches are unhappy with their denominations' increasingly progressive stands on LGBT equality and are organizing to turn back the clock on reproductive rights, LGBT equality, and sexuality education."[140]

Denominational staff have been decreasing as a result of declining national membership numbers (and resulting decreases in national denomination budgets) and policy staff now have many diverse issues in their job portfolios. At this time, none of the surveyed denominations have a person whose sole responsibility is sexual and reproductive rights.

The surveyed denominations differ on the extent of their sexual and reproductive health and justice efforts. Three of the denominations surveyed for this white paper responded that their efforts were stronger in the 1970s than they are now. The UUA and the MCC reported that their efforts are stronger now than in the 1970s. Four reported that their efforts are the same now as they were in the 1970s. More than half say their efforts are about the same now as they were in 2010.

Figure 7. SRH and RJ Efforts by Denomination Since the 1970s

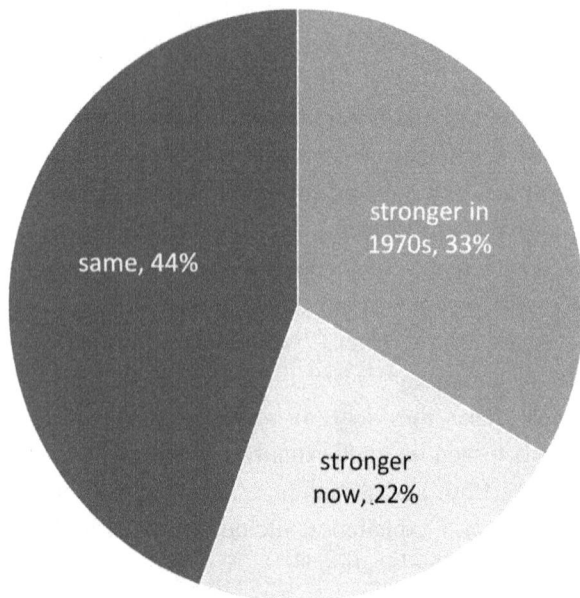

Almost all of the denominations (89 percent) expressed interest in doing more to advocate for sexual and reproductive health and justice. Denominations also articulated several clear needs if they were to increase their efforts: increased staffing (88 percent), financial resources dedicated to SRH and RJ work (88 percent), and congregational materials (44 percent).

When asked about the potential role of faith leaders and people of faith in the sexual and reproductive health and justice movement, denominational leaders spoke to the potential influence of faith voices in public conversations around SRH and RJ issues and their ability to transform and reshape these issues in everyday lives. One respondent suggested that progressive people of faith can "balance the conversation and create space for pro-choice positions." Another offered that faith can help "shift the culture, focus on moral agency of women and on the relationship of health and justice." Another denomination official stated that faith can bring "a more compassionate framework to the public square, connecting the issues to real lives." Many of these denominational officials

believe that faith leaders have the potential to inform the public discourse on issues related to sexual and reproductive health and justice. One denominational official wrote that faith leaders advancing the goals of the SRH and RJ movement are "critical in both pastoral and strategic conversations."

Discussion

Mainline and progressive denominations represent millions of people in the United States and have an important role to play in advocating for sexual and reproductive health and justice. A commitment to sexual health, education, and justice is an opportunity for religious denominations to heal divisions, speak prophetically, and demonstrate pastoral concern for individual struggles with sexuality. Yet only two denominations have increased their work on issues related to sexual and reproductive health and justice in recent years, and many have struggled to maintain their historical commitments to reproductive health. Only the presidents of the most progressive denominations have consistently spoken out on these issues.

Denominations that support sexual and reproductive health and justice can become much more actively involved. Denominations can review and update denomination policies on sexuality education, family planning, and abortion, including adopting a reproductive justice frame and prioritizing reproductive justice as a social justice priority. Denominations are encouraged to make the connection between SRH and RJ and other justice issues that the denomination is already addressing, such as gender equality, poverty, sex trafficking, racism, and economic justice. Denominational public policy offices can designate specific staff to work on sexual and reproductive health and justice issues and to network with secular SRH and RJ organizations.

Religious education departments in all denominations can do more to help congregations implement sexuality education programs. The *Our Whole Lives* program created by the United Church of Christ and the Unitarian Universalist Association is an excellent model of a comprehensive, lifespan sexuality education curriculum that can be adapted to other faith traditions. The Religious Action Center of the Union of Reform Judaism has a program for teenagers called the "L'Taken Social Justice Seminars" in which youth study how to advocate for reproductive health, women's issues, and LGBTQ rights.

More senior denominational officials must speak out on issues related to sexual and reproductive health and justice, including increased financial support for comprehensive sexuality education, family planning, HIV/STI screening and treatment, prenatal care, services for mothers and children, and the repeal of the Hyde and Helms Amendments. In particular, efforts should be made to engage the women who are presidents and bishops of national denominations and movements. In addition, denominations should seek the resources to increase support for the work of extra-denominational organizations committed to women's issues and reproductive health (e.g., Presbyterians Affirming Reproductive Options, Women of the Evangelical Lutheran Church in America, Disciples for Choice, Methodist Federation for Social Action, Unitarian Universalist Women's Federation, etc.)

Denominations can work with religious leaders across the country to respond to state and local attacks on sexual and reproductive health and rights. At the local level, religious leaders must be educated about the connection between sexual justice and social justice. Religious leaders can engage organizations and networks that address racism, poverty, immigration, and other concerns, demonstrating that reproductive and sexual justice cannot be segregated from other justice issues. A more meaningful and faithful public conversation may arise when sexual justice is regarded not just as a political issue but as a pastoral one affecting individuals and families. By focusing on the broader needs of individuals and families, progressive religious leaders may foster a climate of engagement, respectful dialogue, and greater openness and trust.

New strategies must be developed to engage mainstream and progressive religious leaders at the local level. As Sally Steenland wrote in 2011 for the Center for American Progress, organizing is particularly challenging within these communities. She said:

"Mainline and progressive churches tend to be less politically active than their evangelical counterparts, many of which are hubs for pro-life organizing. Mainline ministers are more apt to have congregations with differing views on our issues, as opposed to evangelical churches, which tend to be more ideologically and politically homogenous. Many mainline and progressive clergy are reluctant to get 'too far ahead' of their members or alienate some in the congregation by taking stances on controversial issues. In contrast, evangelical churches have a history of political activism on 'culture war' issues linked to conservative operatives and campaigns. Differences in this 'cultural DNA' between progressive and evangelical churches present challenges for pro-choice advocates seeking faith leaders and places that can be organized."[141]

Efforts must also be made to engage socially progressive evangelicals as well as those who are part of the emerging church. At least one-third of evangelicals support abortion and large majorities support sex education and contraceptive use. Many younger people from evangelical traditions are leaving their churches because of intolerance toward LGBTQ persons[142] and more are engaging in premarital sexual behaviors than in the past.[143] Millennials from evangelical backgrounds may be especially open to opportunities to receive the sex education they have been denied.

Further, progressive evangelical leaders must be educated to understand that economic justice initiatives must also address the reproductive health needs of poor people. During the last decade, although groups such as Faith in Public Life and the Interfaith Alliance have sought to engage evangelical Christians and Roman Catholics on such issues as poverty, climate change, and health care reform, they have largely ignored or excluded sexuality issues. Many of these "progressive" leaders have publicly distanced themselves from abortion or even family planning, ignoring their connections to broader justice issues regarding race, gender, class, poverty, and ecology. As the Religious Institute wrote in 2008, "sexual justice issues are too important to the well-being of the nation to be buried under common ground."[144]

A convening of socially progressive evangelical leaders might be especially timely. Many evangelical leaders have expressed a need to receive sexuality education as pastors, as their education was limited to abstinence-only programs during their high school and college years. The sexual and reproductive health and justice field needs to engage in more sustained discussion about how and under what circumstances it can develop partnerships with religious groups that support contraceptive access but are opposed to abortion.[145]

FAITH-BASED SRH AND RJ ORGANIZATIONS

There are three national US organizations whose primary mission is to work at the intersection of religion with sexual and reproductive health, rights, and justice: Catholics for Choice, the Religious Coalition for Reproductive Choice, and the Religious Institute. RCRC and the Religious Institute use the reproductive justice frame. (The mission statements of the three organizations can be found in the box on page 44.) In addition, three major national organizations with significantly larger budgets—Americans United for Church and State, the Center for American Progress, and the National Council of Jewish Women—have major programmatic initiatives and staff committed to working at the intersection of religion with sexual and reproductive health, rights, and justice.

The Religious Institute created a separate survey to obtain information on these six organizations. Five of the organizations provided a complete response to the survey (see page 60 for a list of respondents who completed the survey). Information from organizations' websites supplement the survey responses.

In total, these six organizations have twenty-two staff persons working on domestic SRH and RJ issues. The combined staffs of RCRC, Catholics for Choice, and the Religious Institute working on domestic sexual and reproductive health and justice is just fourteen people. Among the three larger organizations, between 5 and 10 percent of their total staff address these issues. Not surprisingly, 80 percent of the heads of these organizations responding to the survey indicated that they need increased funding and increased staff in order to have a greater impact. This small number of staff cannot address the large amount of work needed on religion and sexual and reproductive health and justice. Moreover, religious organizations in favor of sexual and reproductive rights have significantly fewer resources than organizations that actively work to oppose them, such as the US Conference of Catholic Bishops, the Family Research Council, Focus on the Family, and other much larger Far Right organizations.

Four of the six faith-based organizations named above have formal clergy networks. Together, they reported having over 14,000 clergy in these networks. All five responding organizations reported that they have a network of people of faith—about 15,000 people are reported to be in these networks.

Each of these organizations has specific strategic goals, target populations, and different organizational strengths. At the same time, there are shared organizational approaches. Five include faith and religion in their strategic plan; conduct specific outreach to faith leaders; publish information on faith issues; do research on religion/faith and issues related to sexual and reproductive health, rights, and justice; engage faith leaders in their public policy efforts; and counter the arguments of the Far Right. Four have religious leaders on their Board of Directors, have a website with dedicated sections on faith issues, and work to counter conscience and refusal clauses. RCRC and the Religious Institute train religious leaders as activists and pastoral care providers. The Religious Institute works directly with congregations and seminaries in creating policies and programs to ensure the sexual health of faith-based institutions.

All of these organizations have assisted secular sexual and reproductive health and justice organizations in engaging religious leaders. All have been asked by colleagues in the SRH and RJ field for help in inviting religious leaders to hearings, rallies, and public witness events and all have written articles or blog posts for secular organizations on the role of faith. Four of the five organizations have been invited to present to the staff of secular organizations in the past five years and two have spoken at the annual meetings of secular organizations. Two reported that they have been asked for assistance in articulating the values-based vision of a secular organization.

The leaders of these faith-based organizations hold different attitudes about the role of faith in the sexual and reproductive health and justice movement than their colleagues at secular organizations. All agree or strongly agree that religious leaders have helped secure reproductive rights in the United States. All also agree or strongly agree that religious leaders have hurt reproductive rights in the United States. They are split on whether religion has done more to hurt than to help. Sixty percent agree that religions have done more to hurt than to help; 40 percent disagree. Unlike their secular colleagues, each of the leaders of these organizations identifies with a faith tradition, and each attends a worship service at least once a month or more.

Not surprisingly, all think that it is important for the sexual and reproductive health and justice field to do more to engage mainstream and progressive people of faith and religious leaders in advocacy efforts. They specifically note the importance of people of faith speaking out in the public square, the importance of changing the public narrative about the morality of reproductive and sexual decisions, the need for secular organizations to advance a values-based vision, the importance of closing the morality/legality divide, and the important role that people of faith can play in public education and advocacy.

These organizations were asked what they felt was currently missing from work on religion. They pointed to the need for more grassroots organizing; more faith-based resources to help people of faith engage in advocacy from a faith-based perspective; more engagement of communities of color, particularly women of color, in faith-based efforts; and more authentic partnerships with secular SRH and RJ organizations.

All of these organizations identified funding as an issue, with four of the five identifying the need for more staff. Four talked about the need for greater collaboration among organizations, and two identified the lack of information and commitment to religious outreach by secular organizations as problematic. Two mentioned the difficulty in motivating supporters at the grassroots level to take action.

Discussion

These faith-based sexual and reproductive health and justice organizations can take the lead in helping frame SRH and RJ as a moral movement and a movement supported by people of faith. The Religious Institute's *Open Letters* can be more widely promoted as moral frameworks for sexuality education, family planning, and abortion. One secular advocate at the colloquium asked for assistance understanding reproductive justice as part of a larger social justice framework. Colloquium participants suggested that the Religious Institute hold a separate colloquium on the morality/legality divide and how to create strategies, consensus, and public narratives on how to close it.

There is a need for even greater partnerships between these six faith-based SRH and RJ organizations and secular SRH and RJ organizations. They can offer training for secular organizations on engaging people of faith, provide secular organizations values-based language, and develop more intensive partnerships with organizations dedicated to reproductive justice that are working with communities of color. There is also a need for more opposition research and strategic development to respond to religious attacks on sexual and reproductive health, rights, and justice.

In the same vein, faith-based SRH and RJ organizations can do more to help denominations increase their commitment to sexual and reproductive health and justice. They can provide training for faith organizations on sexual and reproductive justice; identify and support religious leaders, active lay faith voices, and religious people of color as spokespeople for sexual and reproductive health and justice; and engage chaplains to act as advocates and pastors for SRH and RJ issues.

There is also a need for resources for local congregations, and promotion of the existing resources that the Religious Institute and RCRC have already produced. This includes developing congregational resources for how to talk about SRH and RJ issues, adult study/Bible study group resources, and advocacy materials. There is a need to provide networking opportunities at the state and local level for secular and faith-based SRH and RJ organizations to work together, with a more intensive commitment to support local religious leaders as they combat active religious opposition to sexual and reproductive health and justice, particularly in the South and Midwest.

FOUNDATIONS

As noted in previous sections, the secular organizations, faith-based SRH and RJ organizations, and religious denominations surveyed in preparation for this white paper all stated that they are under-resourced. These organizations do not have enough staff or sufficient programmatic resources to respond to the multiple millions of dollars spent by organizations on the Far Right. Little can be expected to improve until the major foundations supporting sexual and reproductive health and justice also make a commitment to supporting the engagement of religion in the movement.

The Packard Foundation sent the Religious Institute survey to twenty-five foundations that it knew provide funding on SRH and RJ issues. Project officers from fourteen foundations responded to the survey for an overall response rate of 56 percent.

Catholics for Choice's mission is to shape and advance sexual and reproductive ethics that are based on justice, reflect a commitment to women's well-being and respect and affirm the capacity of women and men to make moral decisions about their lives. CFC works in the United States and internationally to ensure that all people have access to safe and affordable reproductive health-care services and to infuse our core values into public policy, community life and Catholic social thinking and teaching.

The **Religious Coalition for Reproductive Choice** is a national community of religious organizations and faithful individuals dedicated to achieving reproductive justice. Through education, organizing and advocacy, RCRC seeks to elevate religious voices wherever faith, policy and our reproductive lives intersect.

The **Religious Institute** advocates for sexual health, education, and justice in faith communities and society. The Religious Institute partners with clergy and other religious leaders, congregations, seminaries, denominations, and secular LGBTQ and reproductive health and justice organizations to promote a progressive religious vision of sexual justice and to help create sexually healthy and responsible religious leaders and faith-based communities.

Fifty-seven percent of these foundations had made grants to organizations working on faith and religion in the United States. One-third (31 percent) had made such grants for international efforts. Six foundations (43 percent) had not funded any faith initiatives within sexual and reproductive health and justice. Of those who had not, half said faith and religion did not fit into their grant priorities, one said their board was not interested in funding religion, and one said they had not seen any organizations worth funding. Of note, none of these six said that they did not believe faith had an important role. Most of the foundations that were not funding SRH and RJ faith initiatives were also not funding faith in other program areas.

Over half of the respondents (54 percent) said that they were likely or very likely to fund a faith or religion project in the future. Twenty-nine percent were "unsure." Despite the lack of significant foundation funding for faith efforts, all of the respondents agreed or strongly agreed that "it is important for the SRH and RJ field to do more to engage mainstream and progressive people of faith and religious leaders in advocacy efforts." Only one of the respondents said that they were somewhat unlikely to fund faith efforts in the future, and none said they were very unlikely.

The foundation respondents were more likely to have a negative attitude about the role of religion in securing reproductive rights compared to the organizations they fund. Three-quarters (77 percent) agree or strongly agree that religions have done more to hurt reproductive rights than secure them in the United States. Only one respondent disagreed with that statement. Three in ten (31 percent) disagreed or strongly disagreed with the statement that religious leaders have helped secure reproductive rights. Only 54 percent agreed that religions have helped secure reproductive rights, compared to 80 percent of leaders in the secular SRH and RJ organizations and 100 percent of the faith-based SRH and RJ organizations. More than nine in ten agreed or strongly agreed that religious leaders have hurt reproductive rights.

More than half (54 percent) of the foundation respondents answered open-ended questions on what more could be done by faith organizations and what role faith could play in the sexual and reproductive health and justice movement. Their suggestions included:

- Moving public attitudes in favor of abortion access
- Collaborating closely with the reproductive justice movement
- Engaging mainstream religious leaders in SRH and RJ advocacy
- Countering religious opposition to contraception, abortion, and sexual behavior among unmarried young adults
- Creating an understanding that reproductive rights are not in conflict with religious beliefs

One respondent wrote:

"Faith plays an important role in the lives of most people in this country, so I don't think we can hope to make a deep change in how people think and act around SRH and RJ without some type of engagement with faith communities, beliefs, leaders, etc. Religious/faith institutions and communities have played important roles in lots of social justice struggles, play an essential role in [advocating for] disenfranchised and marginalized communities across the country, and play an undeniably important role in the American political process, so I see the importance of engaging such institutions/ communities as a matter of necessity from an organizing perspective."

Several foundation respondents mentioned faith organizing as being part of a grassroots movement. One said that "strong grounding in local communities will naturally take us into more engagement of faith communities and leaders, because they are always part of the local infrastructure." Another commented that their likely support for a faith-based initiative would be at a local level. The importance of local engagement is crucial, yet local leaders have told the Religious Institute in focus groups that they need nationally-developed advocacy and education materials specifically for faith communities on sexual and reproductive health and justice in order to become more fully engaged.

This report asks foundations to make a much greater commitment to organizations and programs that articulate the moral framework for the sexual and reproductive health and justice movement, develop religious spokespeople, create faith networks, and engage religious leaders and people of faith. There is a need for foundations to more generously support the core organizations working at the intersection of religion with SRH and RJ with general support grants so that they can resource the secular movement.

Several of the colloquium participants noted that there was a renewed need for strategy building, including how to engage faith. Several suggested a national convening to create an overarching sexual and reproductive health and justice movement strategy, including how religion should be engaged. This could establish the SRH and RJ movement goals for five, ten, and twenty years.

There also may be a need to educate foundations on the role that faith leaders and people of faith can play in advancing SRH and RJ. Presentations at affinity groups or for foundations' Boards of Directors could address the importance of faith, the US faith landscape, the morality/legality divide, current efforts, and opportunities to change the public commitment to sexual and reproductive health and justice.

MEDIA

Media coverage of policy debates too often sets up religion as adversarial to sexual and reproductive health and rights. The media does this on other social justice issues as well, giving conservative and Far Right religious voices far more prominence and visibility than progressive faith voices. From evangelicals to Catholic bishops, opponents have rallied their members and exerted political pressure at the state and national levels, with claims that God and morality are on their side. The media echo these claims by who they choose to feature

in coverage of these issues, resulting in religion being equated in the public mind with opposition to reproductive rights and LGBTQ equality. Too often coverage of public policy issues on sexuality and reproductive health feature a progressive secular leader debating a conservative or even Far Right religious leader, leaving the impression that secular people support sexual and reproductive health and justice and religious people oppose it.

Conservative religious voices dominate the media overall. Conservatives control the country's number one cable news channel (Fox News), newspaper (The Wall Street Journal), talk radio show (Rush Limbaugh), and political news site (Drudge Report).[146] Many of these news organizations and many others are owned by self-professed libertarian Rupert Murdoch. A 2007 report by Media Matters for America found that media coverage of religion over-represents the views of conservative religious voices. The study found that "conservative religious leaders were quoted, mentioned, or interviewed in news stories 2.8 times as often as were progressive religious leaders."[147] On television news, conservative voices appear 3.8 times as often as progressive religious leaders. The report concluded that "it is overwhelmingly conservative leaders that are presented as the voice of religion."[148] It is no wonder that most people in the United States cannot name a national religious leader who is progressive on SRH and RJ issues. Indeed, in the experience of the author of this report, when groups are asked for the name of a progressive religious leader, people are often stumped until someone says, "Pope Francis," without recognition of the Pope's lack of support for sexual and reproductive health issues.

Commentators point to the lack of progressive religious voices in the national media. In 2014, journalist Sarah Posner asked in a Religion Dispatches article, "does the media ignore liberal Christians (or liberal religious people in general)? Does it have—to borrow from the conservative grievance—contempt for them?"[149] She pointed to three examples of recent liberal religious efforts that have been largely ignored by the media: the Moral Mondays movement, the National Gun

Violence Prevention Sabbath Weekend, and the Religious Institute statement signed by forty-seven religious leaders in advance of the Hobby Lobby case. Referring to the Gun Violence Prevention Sabbath, Posner asked "why, as a general matter, these sorts of efforts fail to garner much media attention at all, when conservative Christian events like prayer rallies and denunciations of marriage equality and anti-abortion protests do" receive media attention.[150] Progressive policy analyst Ed Kilgore acknowledges the lopsided religious coverage in the media. He writes, "It kind of makes me crazy when someone appears to assume that only Christian conservatives are authentic religious voices."[151] Yet Kilgore also places some responsibility on progressive religious voices for getting publicity for their perspectives: "the publicity arms of non-conservative religious groups need to do a better job, too," he writes; "the circle of indifference towards the efforts of liberal religious folk is the work of many hands."[152]

A 2015 study of news coverage of contraception-related stories found that national nightly news was more than six times more likely to use a Catholic leader (18 percent) as a source in a story on contraception than they were to use an OB-GYN (3 percent).[153] Government officials and political figures were used 40 percent of the time, the general public was used 26 percent, and media professionals were used 12 percent of the time.[154] As one of the study's authors, Dr. Elizabeth Patton, explains, coverage of contraception "focus[es] on it as a political and social issue, rather than a medical or public health issue."[155] Catholic leaders' voices outweigh not only more progressive religious voices but also the voices of medical professionals. Patton explains that this is because "politicians and some members of the Catholic hierarchy in part drive the news coverage of contraception due to their positions objecting to the ACA mandate."[156] Progressive religious support for the Affordable Care Act (ACA) mandate and for reproductive and sexual justice more broadly, however, receive little coverage.

Conservative religious arguments in the media and the public square require a progressive religious response. The sexual and reproductive health and justice movement must engage religious leaders and faith organizations to respond to attacks by conservatives and the Far Right. Rather than debating religious leaders in the media, secular SRH and RJ organizations should regularly refer the media to faith-based SRH and RJ organizations to suggest progressive religious leaders who can be spokespeople for a particular issue related to sexual and reproductive health and justice.

At the same time, more religious leaders who support sexual and reproductive health and justice need training as spokespeople on SRH and RJ in order to develop their own voice on these issues in the context of their faith traditions. There needs to be a directory of skilled religious speakers and spokespeople in media markets across the country who can address religion and sexuality. The Center for American Progress and Auburn Seminary are working to train local SRH and RJ leaders in more effectively presenting in the media, including identifying new faith media messengers. There needs to be greater emphasis on engaging nationally recognized progressive religious leaders who have a strong media presence. Clergy and religious leaders must also be encouraged to create media opportunities for their support of sexual and reproductive health and justice, such as writing letters to the editor, promoting their advocacy activities, informing their communities and local media about congregational social action events, and more.

Simultaneously, there is a need to educate journalists, editors, and producers from secular, religious, and denominational media on sexual health, education, and justice from a faith perspective. Through one-on-one meetings and national campaigns, the media could learn to represent a plurality of religious voices on SRH and RJ issues. The media need to understand that mainstream and progressive religious voices support sexual and reproductive health and justice from an informed, distinct, and credible religious point of view that contributes to the national conversation. They need to have a directory of people they can call on, and they need to book and quote these progressive faith leaders in their coverage of the news.

CALL TO ACTION

The participants in the National Colloquium on Faith and Sexual and Reproductive Health and Justice created a list of actions for secular SRH and RJ organizations, denominations and religious leaders, faith-based SRH and RJ organizations, and foundations. Although consensus was not reached on all of these ideas (nor are they appropriate for every organization), the colloquium participants affirmed the importance of understanding that sexual and reproductive health and justice organizations should understand and present their cause as a moral movement.

Overall, they urged all who are committed to sexual and reproductive health and justice to:

- Articulate the values-based vision of the SRH and RJ movement
- Create and use values-based language to describe the importance of sexual and reproductive health and justice
- Work to combat cultural stigma around abortion and present abortion as a moral decision
- Develop a culture of storytelling, rooted in real experiences, when discussing SRH and RJ issues
- Shift the cultural conversation from one of judgment to one of empathy and compassion
- Create more convening opportunities for secular and faith leaders to create joint strategies

Further, they emphasized that following the leadership of reproductive justice organizations has the potential to more broadly engage people of faith and faith leaders in issues related to sexual and reproductive health and justice. This will require a commitment of time, money, and resources to develop long-term, non-transactional relationships throughout the movement and also engage with broader struggles for justice, such as the Black Lives Matter and Moral Mondays movements.

SUGGESTED ACTIONS FOR SECULAR SRH AND RJ ORGANIZATIONS

Organizational Commitments

- Include a faith leader on Board of Directors
- Add outreach to faith leaders and people of faith to strategic plan
- Seek funding to develop programs on engaging faith leaders in national, state, and local efforts
- Educate staff and board on why discussing values and faith is important
- Develop staff and board cultural competency about US faith traditions
- Ensure that the workplace is welcoming for people of faith
- Examine anti-religion biases in programs, materials, and website
- Invite religious leaders to speak on relationship between religion and SRH and RJ at annual meetings, conferences, training workshops, and board meetings

Advocacy and Movement Building

- Address values and ethics, in addition to legal arguments, to promote SRH and RJ issues
- Utilize real experiences and storytelling as a way to bridge the morality/legality divide, and encourage compassion, not judgment

- Avoid labeling anti-SRH actions as "religious" or "evangelical" or reinforcing the idea that "all religion is against SRH and RJ"; be specific about the opposition and point out that anti-SRH religious leaders do not speak for all people of faith

- Reference support from the faith community for SRH and RJ issues

- Engage religious leaders and faith organizations to respond to attacks from those opposing SRH and RJ; rather than debating conservative religious leaders in the media, refer to faith-based SRH and RJ organizations to suggest religious leaders who can be spokespeople for particular SRH and RJ issues—conservative religious arguments require a progressive religious response

- Develop partnerships with organizations and religious leaders committed to economic justice

- Create and sustain partnerships with religious organizations, religious leaders, and people of faith

SUGGESTED ACTIONS FOR DENOMINATIONS AND RELIGIOUS LEADERS

Denominations

- Adopt sexual health and education competencies for ordination candidates and continuing education for clergy

- Review and update denominational policies on sexuality education, family planning, and abortion

- Adopt a reproductive justice frame and prioritize reproductive justice as a social justice priority

- Implement denomination-wide training on sexual and reproductive health and justice

- Make the connections between SRH and RJ and other issues that the denomination is already working on, such as gender equality, poverty, trafficking, racism, and economic justice

- Hire designated staff to work on sexual and reproductive health and justice

- Have senior denominational officials speak out on SRH and RJ issues, including comprehensive sexuality education, family planning, HIV/STI screening and treatment, prenatal care, services to mothers and children, and the repeal of the Hyde and Helms Amendments

- Provide support to religious leaders and congregations to resist state-level restrictions on access to reproductive health services, including media templates and strategies for advocating on the local level

- Increase support for the work of extra-denominational organizations committed to women's issues and reproductive health (e.g., Presbyterians Affirming Reproductive Options, Women of the Evangelical Lutheran Church in America, Disciples for Choice, Methodist Federation for Social Action, Unitarian Universalist Women's Federation, etc.)

- Partner with national faith-based SRH and RJ organizations

- Work to eliminate harmful language in official documents that deny rights to LGBTQ people (e.g., marriage equality, ordination, employment discrimination, etc.)

Religious Leaders

- Break the silence about sexuality in congregations

- Commit to working toward ensuring that all congregations are sexually healthy, prophetic, and just

- Make a commitment to engaging sexual and reproductive health and justice within the larger context of social justice

- Develop cultural competency around faith, race, and sexuality issues

- Address sexual justice as a pastoral issue and a political issue

- Educate about the intersections of race, class, gender identity, and sexual orientation

- Encourage existing state and local networks that address racism, poverty, immigration, and economic justice to engage with SRH and RJ issues

SUGGESTED ACTIONS FOR FAITH-BASED SRH AND RJ ORGANIZATIONS

- Promote the *Open Letter* moral frameworks for sexuality education, family planning, and abortion
- Educate about sexual and reproductive justice as part of social justice
- Provide models and methods for using storytelling to advance values-based discussions about SRH and RJ issues
- Provide training for secular organizations on engaging people of faith
- Resource secular organizations with faith voices, faith leaders, and values-based language
- Develop partnerships with organizations dedicated to reproductive justice that are working with communities of color
- Provide training for denominations and other faith organizations on sexual and reproductive justice
- Identify and support religious leaders, active lay voices, and people of color as spokespeople for the movement
- Develop congregational resources for how to talk about SRH and RJ issues
- Develop congregational adult study/Bible study group resources on SRH and RJ issues
- Create relationships with communities of color, supporting their process around SRH and RJ issues and equipping them with the tools they identify to do faith work

- Provide networking opportunities at state and local levels for SRH and RJ and faith organizations to work together
- Commit to supporting local religious leaders as they combat active religious opposition to sexual and reproductive health and justice, particularly in the South and the Midwest
- Develop a proactive strategy to counter religious opposition (opposition research and strategy)

SUGGESTED ACTIONS FOR FOUNDATIONS AND DONORS

Support organizations engaging religion and sexual and reproductive health and justice:
- Fund the three core organizations working at the intersection of faith with SRH and RJ issues with multi-year general support grants
- Provide support to national SRH and RJ organizations for training and resources to do outreach to people of faith and religious leaders

Support long-term movement building:
- Fund gathering(s) designed to create an overarching SRH and RJ movement strategy, including how religion should be engaged
- Support media training for religious leaders supportive of SRH and RJ
- Support education to help media understand faith support of SRH and RJ

Learn about the role faith can play in movements for sexual and reproductive health and justice:
- Invite speakers to meetings of affinity groups and Boards of Directors on role of faith in the SRH and RJ movement, the US faith landscape, the morality/legality divide, effective strategies, etc.

CONCLUDING WORDS

The movement for sexual and reproductive justice is at a critical juncture. Although marriage equality and the Affordable Care Act were affirmed by the Supreme Court in 2015, attacks on access to contraception coverage and abortion services are burgeoning across the country. So-called religious freedom bills and lawsuits to allow employers and providers to deny people their sexual and reproductive rights are proliferating. Discrimination and violence against people of color and transgender people are at particular highs. Too often, discrimination is supported and justified by fundamentalist and conservative religious leaders.

Fifty years ago, religious leaders played a foundational role in securing contraceptive and abortion rights; in more recent years, faith work within the sexual and reproductive health and justice movement has been under-resourced and marginalized. Because organized conservative religion has been a major impediment to sexual and reproductive rights, mainstream and progressive religious leaders must become a much bigger part of efforts to secure those rights. As theologian Daniel Maguire has written, "Religiously nourished illnesses require religious cures."[157]

The morality/legality divide highlighted in this white paper dramatically demonstrates the need for the sexual and reproductive health and justice movement-to re-engage religion. When more than six in ten people in the United States believe that abortion is "morally unacceptable" it is not an overstatement to say that the SRH and RJ movement has lost the hearts of a majority of the US public. Religious engagement cannot be viewed as a luxury or add-on any longer; it must be central to efforts to destigmatize abortion in the United States. The conversation must be changed to help people understand that abortion is a moral decision and that it is the denial of safe, legal, accessible, and affordable services that is immoral.

The sexual and reproductive health and justice movement must develop a stronger relationship with mainline and progressive religious leaders and faith communities. Religious leaders who support reproductive health and rights and have a commitment to the most vulnerable can be found in every state and in every community. They stand ready to be educated and motivated to advocate from their pulpits and in the public square for sexual and reproductive justice.

Faith communities in the United States are ready to embrace gender, sexual, and reproductive justice as essential to ensuring liberty for all. Religious leaders can give voice to the understanding that sexual and reproductive justice are integral to all forms of social justice. As the reproductive justice movement reminds us, all forms of injustice are rooted in oppression. Mainstream and progressive religious leaders are already working to eradicate all forms of oppression that undermine equality and right relationship, including racism, poverty, and economic injustice. With an infusion of resources and a renewed commitment, religious leaders and people of faith can become a mainstay of efforts to secure sexual and reproductive justice as well. Little can be expected to improve until the major foundations and the major secular organizations make a commitment to supporting the engagement of religion in the movement for sexual and reproductive health and justice.

The Religious Institute, its network of religious leaders, and its colleague organizations are poised to help. Together, we can create a future where families in all their diverse forms flourish and all people have the ability and affirmation to make their own moral decisions. So may it be.

APPENDICES

SUGGESTED READING FOR MORE INFORMATION

Background

Asian Communities for Reproductive Justice. "A New Vision for Reproductive Justice: Advancing Our Movement for Reproductive Health, Reproductive Rights and Reproductive Justice." Oakland, 2005. http://strongfamiliesmovement. org/assets/docs/ACRJ-A-New-Vision.pdf.

Balmer, Randall H. *Thy Kingdom Come: How the Religious Right Distorts Faith and Threatens America*. New York: Basic Books, 2007.

Culp-Ressler, Tara. "'God Loves Women Who Have Abortions': The Religious Abortion Advocates that History Forgot." *ThinkProgress* (2014), http:// thinkprogress.org/health/2014/12/16/3601000/ clergy-consultation-service.

Davis, Tom. *Sacred Work: Planned Parenthood and its Clergy Alliances*. New Brunswick, NJ: Rutgers University Press, 2005.

Irvine, Janice. *Talk About Sex: The Battle over Sex Education in the United States*. Berkeley: University of California Press, 2002.

Luna, Zakiya. "From Rights to Justice: Women of Color Changing the Face of US Reproductive Rights Organizing." *Societies without Borders 4*, no. 3 (2009): 343–365, http://www.sistersong.net/ documents/From%20Rights%20to%20Justice%20 by%20Zakiya%20Luna.pdf.

Miller, Patricia. *Good Catholics: The Battle over Abortion in the Catholic Church*. Berkeley: University of California Press, 2014.

Nelson, Jennifer. *More than Medicine: A History of the Feminist Women's Health Movement*. New York: New York University Press, 2015.

Sexuality and Religion

Adler, Rachel. *Engendering Judaism: An Inclusive Theology and Ethics*. Boston: Beacon Press, 2007.

De La Torre, Miguel, Ignacio Castuera, and Lisbeth Meléndez Rivera. *A La Familia: A Conversation about Our Families, the Bible, Sexual Orientation and Gender Identity*. Unid@s, Human Rights Campaign, & National LGBTQ Task Force, 2011. http://www.welcomingresources.org/a_la_familia .pdf.

Ellison, Marvin M. *Making Love Just: Sexual Ethics for Perplexing Times*. Minneapolis: Fortress Press, 2012.

Farley, Margaret. *Just Love: A Framework for Christian Sexual Ethics*. New York: Continuum International Pub. Group, 2006.

Griffin, Horace L. *Their Own Receive Them Not: African American Lesbians and Gays in Black Churches*. Cleveland: The Pilgrim Press, 2006.

Haffner, Debra W., and Timothy Palmer. *Sexuality and Religion 2020: Goals for the Next Decade*. Westport, CT: Religious Institute, 2010.

Maguire, Daniel C. *Sacred Choices: The Right to Contraception and Abortion in Ten World Religions.* Minneapolis: Fortress Press, 2009.

Spong, John Shelby. *The Sins of Scripture: Exposing the Bible's Texts of Hate to Reveal the Love of God.* New York: HarperCollins, 2005.

Tanis, Justin E. *Trans-Gendered: Theology, Ministry, and Communities of Faith.* Cleveland: The Pilgrim Press, 2003.

We are Brave: Building Reproductive Autonomy and Voices for Equity Toolkit: A Manual for Organizations of Color to Champion Abortion Coverage and Reproductive Justice. Portland: Western States Center, 2014.

UPDATES ABOUT RELIGION AND SEXUAL AND REPRODUCTIVE HEALTH AND JUSTICE

To keep up with information about faith in the United States, subscribe to:

- The Public Religion Research Institute's "Morning Buzz": http://publicreligion.org/category/morning-buzz

- Pew Research Center's "Religion and & Public Life" newsletter: http://www.pewforum.org

To keep up with faith and sexual and reproductive health and justice, subscribe to:

- "Faith and Reproductive Justice Weekly" from the Center for American Progress: https://www.americanprogress.org/about/subscribe-faith-reproductive-justice

- Religious Coalition for Reproductive Choice: http://rcrc.org

- Religious Institute: http://www.religiousinstitute.org

- Religion Dispatches: http://religiondispatches.org

- *Conscience* from Catholics for Choice: http://www.catholicsforchoice.org/about/conscience/current

The Religious Institute develops theological frameworks on sexual and reproductive justice issues, with the assistance of the theologians and clergy in its networks. The Open Letters on Abortion and Family Planning are reprinted here. The other Open Letters can be found at www.religiousinstitute.org. Permission is granted to reprint these letters, in part or in full, with attribution to the Religious Institute.

AN OPEN LETTER TO RELIGIOUS LEADERS ON ABORTION AS A MORAL DECISION

As religious leaders, we are committed to supporting people's efforts to achieve spiritual, emotional, and physical well-being, including their reproductive and sexual health. We assist women and families confronted with unintended pregnancies or pregnancies that can no longer be carried to term. We are committed to social justice, mindful of the 46 million women worldwide who have an abortion each year, almost half in dangerous and illegal situations. We seek to create a world where abortion is safe, legal, accessible, and rare.

Millions of people ground their moral commitment to the right to choose in their religious beliefs. While there are strong public health and human rights arguments for supporting the right of women to safe and legal abortion, here we invite you to consider the religious foundations for affirming abortion as a morally justifiable decision.

Affirming Women's Moral Agency

Abortion is always a serious moral decision. It can uphold and protect the life, health, and future of the woman, her partner, and the family.

We affirm women as moral agents who have the capacity, right and responsibility to make the decision as to whether or not abortion is justified in their specific circumstances. That decision is best made when it includes a well-informed conscience, serious reflection, insights from her faith and values, and consultation with a caring partner, family members, and spiritual counselor. Men have a moral obligation to acknowledge and support women's decision-making.

Respect for Life

Our religious traditions affirm that life is sacred. Our faiths celebrate the divinely bestowed blessings of generating life and assuring that life can be sustained and nurtured.

Religious traditions have different beliefs on the value of fetal life, often according greater value as fetal development progresses. Science, medicine, law, and philosophy contribute to this understanding. However, we uphold the teaching of many religious traditions: the health and life of the woman must take precedence over the life of the fetus.

The sanctity of human life is best upheld when we assure that it is not created carelessly. It is precisely because life and parenthood are so precious that no woman should be coerced to carry a pregnancy to term. We support responsible procreation, the widespread availability of contraception, prenatal care and intentional parenting.

Scripture

Scripture neither condemns nor prohibits abortion. It does, however, call us to act compassionately and justly when facing difficult moral decisions. Scriptural commitment to the most marginalized means that pregnancy, childbearing, and abortion should be safe for all women. Scriptural commitment to truth-telling means women must have accurate information as they make their decisions.

Moral Imperative for Access

The ability to choose an abortion should not be compromised by economic, educational, class or marital status, age, race, geographic location or inadequate information. Current measures that limit women's access to abortion services—by denying public funds for low-income women; coercing parental consent and notification as contrasted with providing resources for parental and adolescent counseling; denying international family planning assistance to agencies in developing countries that offer women information about pregnancy options; and banning medical procedures—are punitive and do nothing to promote moral decision-making. When there is a conflict between the conscience of the provider and the woman, the institution delivering the services has an obligation to assure that the woman's conscience and decision will be respected and that she has access to reproductive health care, either directly or through referral. We condemn physical and verbal violence and harassment directed against abortion clinics, their staffs, and their clients.

We must work together to reduce unintended and unwanted pregnancies and address the circumstances that result in the decision to have an abortion. Poverty, social inequities, ignorance, sexism, racism, and unsupportive relationships may render a woman virtually powerless to choose freely. We call for a religious and moral commitment to reproductive health and rights; there must be access to comprehensive sexuality education and contraception, including emergency contraception.

Religious Pluralism

No government committed to human rights and democracy can privilege the teachings of one religion over another. No single religious voice can speak for all faith traditions on abortion, nor should government take sides on religious differences. Women must have the right to apply or reject the principles of their own faith without legal restrictions. We oppose any attempt to make specific religious doctrine concerning abortion the law for all Americans or for the women of the world.

A Call to Religious Leaders

Religious leaders have been in the forefront of the movement for abortion rights for more than fifty years. We call on leaders of all faiths to prepare themselves to offer counsel compassionately, competently, and justly to individuals and families faced with pregnancy decisions. We urge them to:

- Advise and assist adolescent women in involving parents and family members in their decisions, while acknowledging that not every family can offer this support

- Provide age-appropriate faith-based sexuality education that underscores the importance of planned childbearing and responsible sexual decision-making, including abstinence

- Encourage parents to talk openly and honestly about sexuality with their own children

- Counsel women facing pregnancy decisions to reflect, pray, examine their own conscience and faith, and talk with partners and family members

- Support with love to those who choose adoption or termination of their pregnancies, including providing worship opportunities for those who seek them to mourn losses from miscarriages, stillbirths, and abortions

- Provide financial and emotional support for those women who carry their pregnancies to term and provide loving community for them after birth

- Publicly advocate for reproductive rights— including sexuality education, contraception, prenatal care, adoption, and abortion— through sermons, public witness, and involvement in the political process.

In Closing

More than thirty years ago, many religious denominations passed courageous resolutions in support of women's moral agency and their right to a safe and legal abortion. Despite numerous legal challenges and social, scientific and medical advances, we reaffirm this theological commitment: women must be able to make their own moral decisions based on conscience and faith. We call for increased dialog and respectful listening with those who disagree with us. With them, we share the vision of a world where all children are loved and wanted. We renew our own call for relational and reproductive justice for all.

OPEN LETTER TO RELIGIOUS LEADERS ON FAMILY PLANNING

As religious leaders, we are committed to helping all people thrive spiritually, emotionally, and physically, which includes their sexual and reproductive health. Millions of people ground their moral commitment to family planning in their religious beliefs. Most faith traditions accept modern methods of contraception, and support it as a means of saving lives, improving reproductive and public health, enhancing sexuality, and encouraging intentional parenthood. Even within faith groups that limit or prohibit such services, the religious commitment to freedom of conscience allows couples to choose contraception to intentionally create their families. While there are strong public health and human rights arguments for supporting domestic and international family planning programs, here we invite you to consider the religious foundations for affirming safe, affordable, accessible, and comprehensive family planning services.

A Divine Gift

Religious traditions teach that sex and sexuality are divinely bestowed gifts for expressing mutual love, generating life, for companionship, and for pleasure. From a religious point of view, sexual relationships are to be held sacred, and therefore should always be responsible, mutually respectful, pleasurable and loving. The gift of sexuality is violated when it is abused or exploited. Accessible, safe, and effective contraception allows for a fulfilling sexual life while reducing maternal and infant mortality, unintended pregnancies, abortions, and sexually transmitted infections.

Sacredness of Family

Our faith traditions affirm that parenthood is sacred, and therefore should not be entered into lightly nor coerced. Families in their diverse forms are best upheld in environments where there is love and respect, children thrive, and women's welfare is protected. It is unacceptable for society to impose limits on family size or to discriminate against those who choose not to be parents.

Moral Agency

Every individual is a moral agent with the right and responsibility to make their own decisions about procreation, including family size and the spacing of their children. These rights should be accorded equally to all persons regardless of geography, marital status, sexual orientation, gender identity, disability, class, or race. Men and women are equally responsible for contraception and for procreation. Religious institutions have a special role in helping adolescents develop their capacity for moral discernment about relationships, contraception, and procreation.

We believe that all persons should be free to make personal decisions about their families and reproductive lives that are informed by their culture, faith tradition, religious beliefs, conscience, and community. Decisions about which methods to use must be based on informed consent about medical and health risks. The decision to use or not use contraception must always be voluntary.

Scriptural stories honor and welcome diverse families, the care of children, and moral and just decision-making. The scriptural mandate to care for the most marginalized and the most vulnerable calls us to assure access to contraception for all people. The longstanding religious commitment to social and economic justice requires a commitment to reproductive justice.

The commandment to "be fruitful and multiply" is not exclusive to procreation, but also calls individuals to co-create a world characterized by justice and inclusion. Our traditions affirm children as a blessing, not a requirement or an entitlement.

Sacred Texts and Traditions

Our sacred texts are silent on modern contraception. Yet, in the creation stories the world over, the Divine fashions humans intentionally in relationships and families. Family planning is thus a key part of the narrative of many sacred texts.

Moral Imperative to Access

In a just world, all people would have equal access to contraception. The denial of family planning services effectively translates into coercive childbearing and is an insult to human dignity. We affirm a commitment to voluntary family planning services that includes making the full range of safe and effective methods affordable and accessible. The family planning needs of specific populations, such as low-income women, teenagers, immigrants, refugees and LGBT persons, must be addressed with cultural competence.

Governments must respect individual decisions and assure accurate and comprehensive information as well as access to services and supplies. Hospitals and health services, regardless of religious affiliation, must provide or refer to contraceptive services. Services must be offered without regard to sex, age, gender, income, race, religion, marital status, or sexual orientation.

Religious Liberty

No government committed to human rights and democracy can privilege the teachings of one religion over another or deny individuals' religious freedom. Individuals must have the right to accept or reject the principles of their own faith without legal restrictions. No single religious voice can speak for all faith traditions on contraception, nor should government take sides on religious differences. We oppose any attempt to make specific religious doctrine concerning pregnancy, childbirth, or contraception the law of any country in the world. Religious groups themselves must respect the beliefs and values of other faiths, since no single faith can claim final moral authority in domestic or international discourse.

Call to Action

We call on leaders of all faiths to raise a prophetic voice to publicly advocate for universal access to family planning. We urge religious leaders to:

- Educate themselves and their faith communities about sexual and reproductive health and the need for universal access to family planning.
- Compassionately and competently address the needs of their congregants as they make decisions about family planning, contraception, and sexual relationships.
- Contact local family planning providers for referrals, mutual training and support, and encourage those agencies to acknowledge the influence of faith on clients' decisions about contraception.
- Engage in public discourse about the ethical issues involved in research on new methods of contraception.
- Work within their traditions and denominations to make reproductive health a social justice priority.
- Advocate for increased U.S. financial support for domestic and global family planning services through sermons, public witness, and involvement in the political process.

In Closing

Today, as religious leaders, we are called to support universal access to family planning. Religious leaders and people of faith have supported modern methods of contraception since the early 20th century. We resist any political attempts to restrict or deny access to family planning services. Contraception saves lives, promotes human flourishing and advances the common good.

COLLOQUIUM PARTICIPANTS

The following religious leaders and executives of sexual and reproductive health and justice organizations participated in the Religious Institute's National Colloquium on Faith and Sexual and Reproductive Health and Justice in Washington, DC, on April 16, 2015.

Marie Alford-Harkey
Deputy Director
Religious Institute

Rev. Debra W. Haffner
President and CEO
Religious Institute

Jessica Halperin
Witness Ministries Program Associate
Unitarian Universalist Association

Rev. Rob Keithan
Consultant

Drew Konow
Scholar in Residence
Religious Institute

Tamara Kreinin
Director of the Population and
Reproductive Health Program
The David & Lucile Packard Foundation

Rev. Barry Lynn
Executive Director
Americans United for Separation
of Church and State

Carol McDonald
Director of Strategic Partnerships
Planned Parenthood Federation of America

Patricia Miller
Journalist, Author of Good Catholics

Jody Rabhan
Director of Washington Operations
National Council of Jewish Women

Rabbi Dennis Ross
Director
Concerned Clergy for Choice

Shira Saperstein
Principal
ConwayStrategic

Aram A. Schvey
Senior Policy Counsel & Manager
of Special Projects
Center for Reproductive Rights

Monica Raye Simpson
Executive Director
SisterSong

Sally Steenland
Director, Faith and Progressive Policy Initiative
Center for American Progress

Aimée Thorne-Thomsen
Vice President of Strategic Partnerships
Advocates for Youth

Linda Bales Todd
Former Director, Louise and Hugh Moore
Population Project
United Methodist General Board
of Church and Society

Lisa Weiner-Mahfuz
Vice President of Programs and Fund Development
Religious Coalition for Reproductive Choice

SURVEY RESPONDENTS

The following organizations completed surveys for this report.

Secular Organizations

Advocates for Youth

Black Women's Health Imperative

Center for Reproductive Rights

Feminist Majority Foundation

The Guttmacher Institute

NARAL Pro-Choice America (National Abortion and Reproductive Rights Action League)

National Abortion Federation

National Asian Pacific American Women's Forum

National Family Planning & Reproductive Health Association (NFPRHA)

National Latina Institute for Reproductive Health

National Partnership for Women & Families

National Women's Health Network

National Women's Law Center

Physicians for Reproductive Health

Planned Parenthood Federation of America

Reproductive Health Technologies Project

Sexuality Information and Education Council of the United States (SIECUS)

SisterSong

United for Reproductive & Gender Equity (URGE)

Denominations or Denominational Groups

Christian Church (Disciples of Christ)

Evangelical Lutheran Church in America

Metropolitan Community Churches

Muslims for Progressive Values

Presbyterian Church (USA)

Union for Reform Judaism

Unitarian Universalist Association

United Church of Christ

The United Methodist Church

Faith-Based SRH and RJ Related Organizations

Americans United for Separation of Church and State

Center for American Progress

National Council of Jewish Women

Religious Coalition for Reproductive Choice

Religious Institute

Foundations

Buffett Foundation

Compton Foundation

Educational Foundation of America

Foundation for a Just Society

Grove Foundation

Moriah Fund

The Overbrook Foundation

Packard Foundation

The Prospect Hill Foundation

Robert Sterling Clark Foundation

The Summit Foundation

Wellspring Advisors

WestWind Foundation

Wyss Foundation

REFERENCES

1. "The American Values Atlas: Religious Tradition: National," *Public Religion Research Institute*, 2014, http://ava.publicreligion.org/#religious/2014/States/religion/m/national.

2. *U.S. Religious Landscape Survey: Religious Affiliation: Diverse and Dynamic* (Washington, DC: Pew Research Center, 2008), http://religions.pewforum.org/pdf/report-religious-landscape-study-full.pdf, 154.

3. Ibid., "Appendix 2: Detailed Data Tables," http://www.pewforum.org/files/2008/06/report2-religious-landscape-appendix.pdf.

4. "Increasing Racial and Ethnic Diversity within Christianity," *Pew Research Center*, April 30, 2015, http://www.pewforum.org/2015/05/12/americas-changing-religious-landscape/pf_15-05-05_rls2_diversity640px.

5. Debra W. Haffner and James Wagoner, "Vast majority of Americans support sexuality education," *SIECUS Report* 27, no. 6 (1999): 22–23.

6. Robert P. Jones, et al., *The 2012 American Values Survey: How Catholics and the Religiously Unaffiliated Will Shape the 2012 Election and Beyond* (Washington, DC: Public Religion Research Institute, October 2013), http://publicreligion.org/site/wp-content/uploads/2012/10/AVS-2012-Pre-election-Report-for-Web.pdf, 53.

7. "The American Values Atlas: Legality of Abortion: National," *Public Religion Research Institute*, 2014, http://ava.publicreligion.org/#abortion/2014/States/abortion_legality/m/national.

8. See Tom Davis, *Sacred Work: Planned Parenthood and Its Clergy Alliances* (New Brunswick, NJ: Rutgers University Press, 2005).

9. Robert P. Jones, et al. *A Shifting Landscape: A Decade of Change in American Attitudes about Same-Sex Marriage and LGBT Issues* (Washington, DC: Public Religion Research Institute, February 2014), http://publicreligion.org/site/wp-content/uploads/2014/02/2014.LGBT_REPORT.pdf.

10. "Politico on New Poll By NARAL Pro-Choice America Showing 7 in 10 Americans Support Legal Abortion," *NARAL Pro-Choice America*, August 18, 2014, http://www.prochoiceamerica.org/elections/elections-press-releases/2014/20140818_politico_7in10_poll.html. On the question of morality, see "Abortion Viewed in Moral Terms: Fewer See Stem Cell Research and IVF as Moral Issues," Pew Research Center, August 15, 2013, http://www.pewforum.org/2013/08/15/abortion-viewed-in-moral-terms. See also Jones et al., The 2012 American Values Survey, 50; and Jones et al., A Shifting Landscape, 42.

11. Excerpted from "What is RJ?" at http://www.sistersong.net.

12. *We Are Brave: Building Reproductive Autonomy and Voices for Equity Toolkit: A Manual for Organizations of Color to Champion Abortion Coverage and Reproductive Justice* (Portland: Western States Center, 2014), 31.

13. Marvin M. Ellison. *Making Love Just: Sexual Ethics for Perplexing Times* (Minneapolis: Fortress Press, 2012), 6.

14. "Social Justice" in Robert Wuthnow (ed.), *Encyclopedia of Politics and Religion* (Washington, D.C.: CQ Press, 2007), 778–866.

15. "The American Values Atlas: Religious Tradition: National," *Public Religion Research Institute*.

16. See "Fast Facts about American Religion." *Hartford Institute for Religion Research, accessed May 11, 2015, http://hirr.hartsem.edu/research/fastfacts/fast_facts.html.

17. *U.S. Religious Landscape Survey*, 177.

18. Ibid., 162.

19. Ibid., 154.

20. Ibid.

21. "The American Values Atlas: Religious Tradition: National," *Public Religion Research Institute*.

22. Ibid.

23. *U.S. Religious Landscape Survey*, 5.

24. "The American Values Atlas: Religious Tradition: National," *Public Religion Research Institute*. The United Methodist Church, the Evangelical Lutheran Church in America, the Presbyterian Church USA, American Baptist Churches USA, the Episcopal Church, the United

Church of Christ, and Christian Church (Disciples of Christ) comprise the large majority of mainline Protestantism (although some accounts consider other, smaller groups like Quakers, Moravians, and the Reformed Church in America to be mainline as well).

25. "The American Values Atlas: Religious Tradition: National," *Public Religion Research Institute.*

26. Ibid.

27. "State of the Bible 2015," *American Bible Society,* February 2015, www.state-of-the-Bible-2015-report.pdf, 13, 11.

28. Ibid., 25–26.

29. The American Values Atlas: Religious Tradition: National," *Public Religion Research Institute.*

30. "The American Values Atlas: Religious Tradition: National," *Public Religion Research Institute. For the purposes of this report, the Southern region of the United States is defined as including the states of Alabama, Arkansas, Delaware, Florida, Georgia, Kentucky, Louisiana, Mississippi, North Carolina, Oklahoma, South Carolina, Tennessee, Texas, Virginia, and West Virginia. This definition follows PRRI.*

31. "How Religious Is Your State?" *Pew Research Center, December 21, 2009, http://www.pewforum. org/2009/12/21/how-religious-is-your-state.*

32. "Appendix 2: Detailed Data Tables" in *U.S. Religious Landscape Survey.*

33. The other most religious state is Utah. Frank Newport, "Mississippi Most Religious State, Vermont Least Religious: Average Religiousness of States Continues to Range Widely," *Gallup, February 3, 2014, http:// www.gallup.com/poll/167267/ mississippi-religious-vermont-least-religious-state.aspx; and* "How Religious Is Your State?"

34. "State of the Bible 2015," *American Bible Society,* 13.

35. *U.S. Religious Landscape Survey,* 18.

36. Data compiled from National Opinion Research Center, *General Social Surveys 1972– 2014: Cumulative Codebook: March 2015 (Chicago: University of Chicago, 2015).*

37. Ibid.

38. "America's Changing Religious Landscape." *Pew Research Center, May 15, 2015, http:// www.pewforum.org/2015/05/12/ americas-changing-religious-landscape.*

39. See "America's Changing Religious Landscape, " *Pew Research Center. And on Southern evangelicals specifically see Robert P. Jones, "Southern Evangelicals: Dwindling," The Atlantic, October 17, 2014, www.theatlantic.com/politics/ archive/2014/10/-the-shrinking-evangelical-voter-pool/381560.*

40. Data compiled from National Opinion Research Center, *General Social Surveys 1972– 2014.*

41. "America's Changing Religious Landscape," *Pew Research Center,* 33.

42. Ibid.

43. Data compiled from National Opinion Research Center, *General Social Surveys 1972– 2014.*

44. Ibid.

45. Ibid.

46. Ibid.

47. "'Nones' on the Rise," *Pew Research Center, October 9, 2012, http://www.pewforum. org/2012/10/09/nones-on-the-rise.*

48. "U.S. Religious Landscape Survey: Religious Beliefs and Practices," *Pew Research Center, June 1, 2008, http://www. pewforum.org/2008/06/01/ u-s-religious-landscape-survey-religious-beliefs-and-practices.*

49. *Sex Education in America: General Public/Parents Survey, National Public Radio/ Kaiser Family Foundation/ Kennedy School of Government, January 2004, https:// kaiserfamilyfoundation.files. wordpress.com/2013/01/sex-education-in-america-general-public-parents-survey-toplines .pdf,* 5.

50. Robert P. Jones, et al., *Committed to Availability, Conflicted about Morality: What the Millennial Generation Tells Us about the Future of the Abortion Debate and the Culture Wars (Washington, DC: Public Religion Research Institute, June 2011), http://publicreligion.org/ site/wp-content/uploads/2011/06/ Millenials-Abortion-and-Religion-Survey-Report.pdf,* 18.

51. Debra W. Haffner and James Wagoner, "Vast majority of Americans support sexuality education."

52. Robert P. Jones, et al., *The 2012 American Values Survey,* 53.

53. "Religious, Partisan and Gender Differences: Public Divided over Birth Control Insurance Mandate," *Pew Research Center, February 14, 2012,* 8.

54. Rachel K. Jones and Joerg Dreweke, "Countering Conventional Wisdom: New Evidence on Religion and Contraceptive Use" (New York: Guttmacher Institute, 2011), https://www.guttmacher .org/pubs/Religion-and-Contraceptive-Use.pdf.

55. Ibid.

56. "The American Values Atlas: Legality of Abortion: National," *Public Religion Research Institute.*

57. "Politico on New Poll By NARAL Pro-Choice America Showing 7 in 10 Americans Support Legal Abortion," *NARAL Pro-Choice America.*

58. Rachel K. Jones and Joerg Dreweke, "Countering Conventional Wisdom: New Evidence on Religion and

Contraceptive Use."

59. "The American Values Atlas: Availability of Abortion: National," *Public Religion Research Institute*, 2014, http://ava.publicreligion.org/#abortion/2014/States/abortion_availability/m/national.

60. "The American Values Atlas: Legality of Abortion: National," *Public Religion Research Institute*.

61. "Public Opinion on Abortion," *Pew Research Religion & Public Life Project*, July 2013, http://features.pewforum.org/abortion-slideshow/slide3.php.

62. "Section 3: Social & Political Issues," *Pew Research Center*, September 22, 2014, http://www.pewforum.org/2014/09/22/section-3-social-political-issues.

63. "Poll: Latino Voters Hold Compassionate Views on Abortion," *Lake Research Partners*, 2011, http://latinainstitute.org/sites/default/files/LatinoAbortionAttitudesPolling.pdf.

64. "Section 3: Social & Political Issues," *Pew Research Center*.

65. "Public Opinion on Abortion," *Pew Research Religion & Public Life Project*; "Section 3: Social & Political Issues," *Pew Research Center*.

66. "Abortion Viewed in Moral Terms: Fewer See Stem Cell Research and IVF as Moral Issues," *Pew Research Center*. *See also 51 percent in Robert P. Jones, et al., The 2012 American Values Survey. See also 54 percent in Robert P. Jones, et al., A Shifting Landscape, 42.*

67. Robert P. Jones, et al., *A Shifting Landscape*, 45.

68. Robert P. Jones, et al., *The 2012 American Values Survey*, 45.

69. "Abortion Viewed in Moral Terms: Fewer See Stem Cell Research and IVF as Moral Issues," *Pew Research Center*.

70. "Politico on New Poll By NARAL Pro-Choice America Showing 7 in 10 Americans Support Legal Abortion," *NARAL Pro-Choice America*.

71. Robert P. Jones, et al., *A Shifting Landscape*, 42.

72. Robert P. Jones, et al., *The 2012 American Values Survey*, 50–51.

73. Robert P. Jones, et al., *A Shifting Landscape*, 42.

74. Rachel K. Jones and Megan L. Kavanaugh, et al., "Changes in Abortion Rates between 2000 and 2008 and Lifetime Incidence of Abortion," *Obstetrics & Gynecology 117*, no. 6 (2011):1358–1366.

75. Rachel K. Jones, et al., "Characteristics of U.S. Abortion Patients, 2008" (New York: Guttmacher Institute, 2010), 9.

76. Ibid.

77. Rachel K. Jones and Megan L. Kavanaugh, "Changes in Abortion Rates between 2000 and 2008 and Lifetime Incidence of Abortion."

78. Ibid.

79. Robert P. Jones, et al., *A Shifting Landscape*, 42.

80. Rachel K. Jones and Megan L. Kavanaugh, "Changes in Abortion Rates between 2000 and 2008 and Lifetime Incidence of Abortion."

81. "*Roe v. Wade* at 40: Most Oppose Overturning Abortion Decision," *Pew Research Center*, January 16, 2013, http://www.pewforum.org/2013/01/16/roe-v-wade-at-40.

82. Ibid.

83. Robert P. Jones, et al., *LGBT Issues and Trends Survey* (Washington, DC: Public Religion Research Institute, February 2014), http://publicreligion.org/site/wp-content/uploads/2014/02/2014-LGBT-Topline-FINAL.pdf.

84. Ibid.

85. On unaffiliated vote, see: Juhem Navarro-Rivera, "The Evolution of the Religiously Unaffiliated Vote, 1980–2008," *Public Religion Research Institute*, October 26, 2012, http://publicreligion.org/2012/10/the-evolution-of-the-religiously-unaffiliated-vote-1980-2008/#.VV3i2PlVhBc.

86. "Public Sees Religion's Influence Waning: Section 2: The Religious Landscape of the 2014 Elections," *Pew Research Center*, September 22, 2014, http://www.pewforum.org/2014/09/22/section-2-the-religious-landscape-of-the-2014-elections.

87. Robert P. Jones, et al., *A Shifting Landscape*.

88. "The American Values Atlas: Legality of Abortion: National," *Public Religion Research Institute*.

89. Robert P. Jones, et al., *A Shifting Landscape*, 45.

90. "Politico on New Poll By NARAL Pro-Choice America Showing 7 in 10 Americans Support Legal Abortion," *NARAL Pro-Choice America*.

91. Robert P. Jones, et al., *Religion, Values, & Experiences: Black and Hispanic American Attitudes on Abortion and Reproductive Issues* (Washington, DC: Public Religion Research Institute, July 2012), http://publicreligion.org/site/wp-content/uploads/2012/07/Reproductive-Survey-Report.pdf.

92. Quoted in *We Are Brave*, 69.

93. See Tom Davis, "Chapter 4: The 1958 Battle Over the New York City Hospitals" in *Sacred Work*.

94. "Our Whole Lives: Lifespan Sexuality Education," *Unitarian Universalist Association*, www.uua.org/re/owl.

95. Tara Culp-Ressler, "'God Loves Women Who Have Abortions': The Religious Abortion Advocates that History Forgot," *ThinkProgress*, December 16, 2014, http://thinkprogress.org/health/2014/12/16/3601000/clergy-consultation-service/.

96. For full text of the resolution, see "Birth Control," *Central Conference of American Rabbis*, http://ccarnet.org/rabbis-speak/resolutions/all/birth-control-1889-1972.

97. For full text of the resolution, see "Universalists Back Birth Control Idea," *New York Times*, October 24, 1929, http://query.nytimes.com/gst/abstract.html?res=9B0DE0D91639E03ABC4D51DFB6678382639EDE.

98. For full text of the resolution, see *The Lambeth Conference: Resolutions Archive from 1930*, http://www.anglicancommunion.org/media/127734/1930.pdf?language=English, 7.

99. For full text of the report, see "Protestants Endorse Birth Control," *Birth Control Review* XV, no. 4 (April 1931), http://birthcontrolreview.net/Birth%20Control%20Review/1931-04%20April.pdf.

100. For full text of the resolution, see "Birth Control Literature: Resolutions and Statements: 1935," https://www.wrj.org/social-justice/resolutions-statements/most-important/birth-control.

101. Pius XI, "Casti Connubii," *Libreria Editrice Vaticana*, December 31, 1930, http://w2.vatican.va/content/pius-xi/en/encyclicals/documents/hf_p-xi_enc_31121930_casti-connubii.html.

102. Paul VI, "Humanae Vitae," *Libreria Editrice Vaticana*, July 25, 1968, http://w2.vatican.va/content/paul-vi/en/encyclicals/documents/hf_p-vi_enc_25071968_humanae-vitae.html.

103. Patricia Miller, *Good Catholics: The Battle over Abortion in the Catholic Church* (Berkeley: University of California Press, 2014), 66–67.

104. Randall Balmer, "The Real Origins of the Religious Right: They'll Tell You it was Abortion. Sorry, the Historical Record's Clear: It was Segregation," *Politico*, May 27, 2014, http://www.politico.com/magazine/story/2014/05/religious-right-real-origins-107133_full.html#.VVodrvlVhBd.

105. Quoted in Randall Balmer, "The Real Origins of the Religious Right."

106. Randall Balmer, "The Real Origins of the Religious Right."

107. Ibid.

108. "Catholic Health Care Update: The Facts about Catholic Health Care in the United States," *Catholics for a Free Choice*, September 2005, http://www.catholicsforchoice.org/topics/healthcare/documents/2005factsaboutcatholichealthcare_000.pdf.

109. Americans United for the Separation of Church and State, *Frequently Asked Questions About RFRA and Hobby Lobby* (Washington, DC: Americans United for Separation of Church and State, 2015), 1–2.

110. Ibid., 2.

111. Ibid., 4.

112. "Open Letter to Religious Leaders on Family Planning," *Religious Institute*, 2012, http://www.religiousinstitute.org/wp-content/uploads/2014/02/Open-Letter-on-Family-Planning-with-endorsers-2014.pdf.

113. For full text of the brief, see "Brief of Religious Organizations," http://www.becketfund.org/wp-content/uploads/2014/01/Nos.-13-354-13-356tsacBriefofReligiousOrganizations.pdf.

114. See Tara Culp-Ressler, "'Religious Freedom' Laws Threaten to Roll Back Women's Access to Basic Health Care," *ThinkProgress*, April 14, 2015, http://thinkprogress.org/health/2015/04/14/3646936/religious-freedom-reproductive-rights.

115. Americans United for the Separation of Church and State, *Frequently Asked Questions About RFRA and Hobby Lobby*, 1–2.

116. "London Declaration of Prochoice Principles," *Catholics for Choice*, September 2012.

117. "National Religious Leaders Affirm Access to Birth Control in Advance of SCOTUS Hearing," *Religion News Service*, March 18, 2014, http://pressreleases.religionnews.com/2014/03/18/national-religious-leaders-affirm-access-birth-control-advance-scotus-hearing/#sthash.4XFuxzow.dpuf.

118. "Religion and Spirituality," *Advocates for Youth*, http://www.advocatesforyouth.org/religion-and-spirituality.

119. "The Muslim Youth Project," *Advocates for Youth*, http://www.advocatesforyouth.org/about-us/programs-and-initiatives/345?task=view.

120. "Using Religion to Discriminate," *ACLU: American Civil Liberties Union*, https://www.aclu.org/feature/using-religion-discriminate.

121. "Mission, Vision, & Values," *National Latina Institute for Reproductive Health*, http://www.latinainstitute.org/en/mission-vision-values-0.

122. Lindsay Beyerstein, "Abortion without Apology: A Prescription for Getting Pro-Choice Groove Back," *The American Prospect*, October 14, 2014, http://prospect.org/article/abortion-without-apology-prescription-getting-

pro-choice-groove-back.

123. "Unapologetic, Native, New Yorker," *Abortion Looks Like*, *http://abortionlookslike.tumblr.com/post/115871575422/unapologetic-native-new-yorker*.

124. "Abortion Viewed in Moral Terms: Fewer See Stem Cell Research and IVF as Moral Issues," *Pew Research Center*.

125. Ibid.

126. "1 in 3 Women Will Have an Abortion in her Lifetime. These are Our Stories," *Advocates for Youth*, *www.1in3campaign.org/en*.

127. Catholics for Choice, British Pregnancy Advisory Service, et al., "Lisbon, 2014: An International Summit on Reproductive Choice," 2015, http://www.catholicsforchoice.org/topics/abortion/documents/2015Lisbonpublication.pdf, 41.

128. "UUA, UUWF Presidents Commemorate 40th Anniversary of *Roe v. Wade* Decision," *Unitarian Universalist Association*, *January 22, 2013, http://www.uua.org/news/pressroom/pressreleases/281877.shtml*.

129. "Interfaith Celebration Honoring the 40th Anniversary of *Roe v Wade and the Founding of the Religious Coalition for Reproductive Choice*," Metropolitan Community Churches, *January 17, 2013, http://mccchurch.org/interfaith-celebration-honoring-the-40th-anniversary-of-roe-v-wade-and-the-founding-of-the-religious-coalition-for-reproductive-choice*.

130. "UMC Support: Responsible Parenthood (#2025 2012 BOR)," *Healthy Families Healthy Planet*, 2012, *http://umchealthyfamilies.org/umc-support/um-resolutions/responsible-parenthood-2025-2012-bor*.

131. "Federal Legislation for Choice: 1993 General Resolution," *Unitarian Universalist Association*, 1993, *http://www.uua.org/statements/federal-legislation-choice*.

132. Ibid.

133. "Proactive Prevention: Seeking Common Ground on the Issue of Abortion," *Christian Church (Disciples in Christ)*, *July 2007, http://disciples.org/Portals/0/PDF/ga/pastassemblies/2007/resolutions/0725.pdf*.

134. "Reaffirm General Convention Statement on Childbirth and Abortion," *The Archives of the Episcopal Church*, 1994, *http://www.episcopalarchives.org/cgi-bin/acts/acts_resolution.pl?resolution=1994-A054*.

135. Ibid.

136. United Church of Christ, *General Synod Statements and Resolutions Regarding Freedom of Choice, http://d3n8a8pro7vhmx.cloudfront.net/unitedchurchofchrist/legacy_url/2038/GS-Resolutions-Freedon-of-Choice.pdf?1418425637*, 11.

137. "Statement of Faith on Women's Reproductive Health, Rights, and Justice," *Metropolitan Community Churches*, March 20, 2013, *http://mccchurch.org/statement-of-faith-on-womens-reproductive-health-rights-and-justice*.

138. "Reproductive Justice," *Unitarian Universality Association, http://www.uua.org/reproductive*.

139. "Reproductive Justice: 2015 Statement of Conscience," *Unitarian Universalist Association*, 2015, *http://www.uua.org/statements/reproductive-justice*.

140. Sally Steenland, "Faith and Sexual Justice: Assessing the Landscape of Sexual and Reproductive Rights and Justice Work," *Center for American Progress, September 30, 2011.

141. Ibid.

142. David Kinnaman, *You Lost Me: Why Young Christians are Leaving Church...and Rethinking Faith (Grand Rapids: Baker Books, 2011)*.

143. A 2012 video from the National Association of Evangelicals puts this at 80 percent. See Adele Banks, "With High Premarital Sex and Abortion Rates, Evangelicals Say it's Time to Talk about Sex," *Huffington Post/Religion New Service, April 23, 2012, http://www.huffingtonpost.com/2012/04/23/evangelicals-sex-frank-talk_n_1443062.html?*.

144. Debra Haffner and Timothy Palmer, "Toward a Theology of Sexual Justice," in *Dispatches from the Religious Left*, ed. *Frederick Clarkson (Brooklyn: IG Publishing, 2008), 90*.

145. This conversation has already begun in many different areas of the sexual and reproductive health and justice movement. *Conscience Magazine dedicated an entire issue to the question. See Conscience XXXV, no. 3, 2014, http://www.catholicsforchoice.org/about/conscience/current/documents/Conscience2014-3.pdf*.

146. Dylan Byers, "What Liberal Mainstream Media?" *Politico, September 18, 2013, http://www.politico.com/blogs/media/2013/09/what-liberal-mainstream-media-172952.html*.

147. "Left Behind: The Skewed Representation of Religion in Major News Media." *Media Matters for America*, July 2007, *http://mediamatters.org/research/leftbehind*.

148. Ibid.

149. Sarah Posner, "Is Coverage

of Liberal Religion a Media Fail?" *Religion Dispatches, March 18, 2014, http://religiondispatches.org/is-coverage-of-liberal-religion-a-media-fail.*

150. Sarah Posner, "More Thoughts on Media Coverage of Liberal Religion," *Religion Dispatches, March 18, 2014, http://religiondispatches.org/more-thoughts-on-media-coverage-of-liberal-religion.*

151. Quoted in Sarah Posner, "Is Coverage of Liberal Religion a Media Fail?"

152. Ibid.

153. Jen Gunter, "Nightly News Speaks More to Catholic Church about Contraception than OB/GYNs. A Lot More," *Dr. Jen Gunter: Wielding the Lasso of Truth, May 5, 2014, https://drjengunter.wordpress.com/2015/05/05/nightly-news-speaks-more-to-catholic-church-about-contraception-than-obgyns-a-lot-more.*

154. Patricia Miller, "Nightly News Turns to Bishops about Contraception More Often than Docs," *Religion Dispatches, May 8, 2015, http://religiondispatches.org/nightly-news-turns-to-bishops-about-contraception-more-often-than-docs.*

155. Ibid.

156. Ibid.

157. Daniel Maguire, "Violence against Women: Roots and Cures in World Religions," *The Religious Consultation on Population,* http://www.religiousconsultation.org/violence_vs_women_roots_and_cures_in_world_religions.htm.

ABOUT RELIGIOUS INSTITUTE

Founded in 2001, the Religious Institute is a national, multifaith organization dedicated to promoting sexual health, education, and justice in faith communities and society. The Religious Institute partners with clergy and congregations, denominations, seminaries, national advocacy organizations, and sexual and reproductive health organizations to promote:

- Sexually healthy faith communities
- Full equality of women and lesbian, gay, bisexual, transgender, and queer persons in congregations and communities
- Marriage equality
- Comprehensive sexuality education
- Reproductive justice
- A responsible approach to adolescent sexuality
- Sexual abuse prevention
- HIV/AIDS education and prevention
- Global sexual health

The mission of the Religious Institute is to develop a new understanding of the relationship between religion and sexuality. This mission involves:

- Developing and supporting a network of clergy, religious educators, theologians, ethicists, and other religious leaders committed to sexual justice.
- Building the capacity of religious institutions and clergy to provide sexuality education within the context of their faith traditions.
- Helping congregations, seminaries, and denominations to become sexually healthy faith communities.
- Educating the public and policymakers about a progressive religious vision of sexual morality, justice, and healing.

The Religious Institute's network includes more than 15,000 religious leaders and people of faith from more than 70 faith traditions who are committed to sexual health, education, and justice in faith communities and society.

NOTES